RADIOGRAPHIC POSITIONING

and

Related Anatomy

Workbook and Laboratory Manual

VOLUME I   Chapters 1-13

RADIOGRAPHIC POSITIONING and
Related Anatomy
Workbook and Laboratory Manual

THIRD EDITION

Kenneth L. Bontrager, M.A., RT (R)

Mosby

St. Louis Baltimore Boston Chicago London Madrid Philadelphia Sydney Toronto

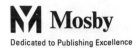

Mosby
Dedicated to Publishing Excellence

Data Entry and Page Layout:	Troy Bontrager
	Mary Lou Bontrager
Illustrations:	Debra Ravin
	Sally Schmitt
	Joan Lapre
	Don O'Connor

Printed in the United States of America
Composition by Mosby Electronic Production, St. Louis
Printing/binding by Plus Communications

Mosby–Year Book, Inc.
11830 Westline Industrial Drive
St. Louis, Missouri 63146

International Standard Book Number 0-8016-8057-3

93 94 95 96   MS/PC   9 8 7 6 5 4 3 2 1

Acknowledgments

I am pleased to acknowledge and recognize those persons who have made significant contributions and provided much support and encouragement during the planning and preparation of the new third edition of this student workbook and laboratory manual.

The following persons reviewed drafts of proposed format changes and made suggestions in addition to reviewing and proofing each chapter prior to final preparation. These are:

Eugene Frank, RT, Mayo Clinic, Rochester, MN
David Hall, RT, Broward Community College, Davies, FL
Fred Price, RT, Garland Community College, Hot Springs National Park, AR
Dennis Spragg, RT, Lima Technical College, Lima, OH

I also want to thank those contributing authors who submitted information that could be incorporated into these specific chapters. As identified under the specific chapters to which they contributed, these are:

Nancy Dickerson, RT, Mayo Clinic, Rochester, MN
Eugene Frank, RT, Mayo Clinic, Rochester, MN
John Lampignano, RT, Gateway Community College, Phoenix, AZ
Kathy Martensen, RT, University of Iowa Hospitals and Clinics, Iowa City, IA
Joan Radke, RT, University of Iowa Hospitals and Clinics, Iowa City, IA

I also want to acknowledge and thank **Barry Anthony**, RT, for his significant contributions to the first and second editions of this workbook.

Last and most important to me are the acknowledgments and thanks to my wife **Mary Lou** and to our son **Troy** for their major contributions to this work through their expert typing and computer skills. I thank you Troy for taking time between your college studies and graduate school to help me with this major project. Once again I also thank you Mary Lou for your support and your continuing major contributions to my writing projects.

KLB

Preface

The success of the first two editions of this workbook and the accompanying Radiographic Anatomy and Positioning audio-visuals is evidenced by the high percentage of schools of Radiologic Technology throughout the United States and Canada that have been using these materials for over twenty years.

These workbooks have been widely recognized as an effective learning tool even without the audio-visuals. Therefore with the completion of the expanded third edition textbook, these workbooks were also revised and expanded to be more effective.

The laboratory exercises have been expanded to include more positioning exercises as well as film critique and evaluation exercises based on specific evaluation criteria. Thus this new third edition has become a combination workbook and laboratory manual.

The revised format of this new edition is effective when used with the textbook alone or with the combination of textbook and audio-visuals. Therefore the self-paced learning format advantages are retained. This format makes optimal use of the instructor's time by allowing students to repeat sections as needed to master the material through individual study prior to taking the final evaluation exam. Thus students are better prepared for their clinical experience because they have all reached a predetermined competency level in their positioning knowledge and skills.

Relationship of Workbook and Laboratory Manual to Textbook

This third edition of the student workbook and laboratory manual is organized to be in complete agreement with the third edition of the Bontrager textbook. The workbook and laboratory manual is divided into 2 volumes. Each of the 25 chapters in the textbook has an equivalent chapter in these workbook/lab manuals to reinforce and supplement the information presented. This includes both the study of anatomy and the related positioning, including film critique and evaluation of specific body parts as described in each chapter.

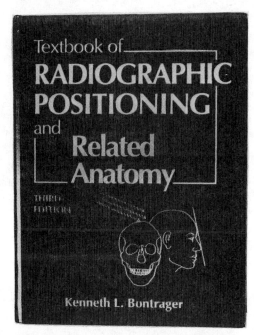

The most effective use of this workbook/laboratory manual is for the student to complete the chapter exercises immediately after reading and studying the corresponding chapter in the textbook. To make the most effective and best use of instructor's time, this study should be done prior to the classroom presentation. In this way the instructor can spend more time in both the classroom and laboratory on problem areas and less time on the fundamentals which the students should have learned from their individual study using the textbook combined with these workbook/lab manuals.

This workbook/laboratory manual can also be used with other textbooks and resource materials, such as the Bontrager/Anthony Radiographic Anatomy and Positioning audio-visual series, provided that the contents of each chapter in this workbook is closely coordinated with the information in the other resource materials.

Kenneth L. Bontrager

Contents

VOLUME I

VOLUME II

Student Instructions

Reading these instructions is VITALLY IMPORTANT if you are to receive maximum benefit from this workbook.

If you will take the time to read the following information, you will discover how correct use of this self-paced learning method will help you master the knowledge and skills of radiographic anatomy and positioning.

This course becomes the core or the central course of all your studies and your work as a radiographer. Therefore **this is one course each of you must master.** You cannot become a proficient radiographer by only marginally passing this course. Therefore please read these instructions carefully **before** beginning your study of Chapter 1.

Rationale

The rationale in each chapter should help you understand **why** you need to learn this material and **how you will use it** as a student and a future radiologic technologist.

Objectives

The list of objectives should be studied carefully so that you will understand what you must know and be able to do when you complete each chapter.

Prerequisites and Recommended Supplementary References

The prerequisites for this study describe what minimum level of reading and understanding is required to master this series. The specific prerequisites for each chapter are listed.

The supplementary references are provided to allow you additional resources for more information on the material covered in each of these chapters. They are listed in a suggested order of importance. The specific pages are included to help you look up this information more readily. The importance of these references will vary depending on your background knowledge and experience but it is suggested that you look up and review the information in at least one of these references.

Learning Exercises

These exercises will be the focal point of this workbook/laboratory manual. Using them correctly will reinforce and help you learn and remember the important information as presented in each chapter of the textbook and/or audio-visuals. For you to receive the maximum benefit from these exercises, follow the correct order of activities as outlined below.

Combination of textbook and/or audio-visual presentation used in correlation with student workbook and laboratory manual.

Step 1. **Textbook:** Carefully read and learn the anatomy in Part I of the chapter being studied. Include the anatomy reviews on labeled radiographs provided in each chapter of the textbook.

Audio-visuals if available: Complete the audio-visual presentation for Part I covering the anatomy of that chapter or unit. Do *not* write in the workbook during the audio-visual presentation.

Step 2. **Workbook:** Complete Part I of the review exercises. Do not look up the answers in the textbook or look at the answer sheet until you have completed answering as many of the questions as you can. Only then look in the textbook and/or at the answer sheet and correct or complete those questions you missed.

If you missed more than the suggested minimum for each exercise, you should go back and review that section again in the textbook and the audio-visuals before continuing to the next section.

Step 3. **Textbook:** Carefully study Part II on radiographic positioning in the textbook. Take note of the general positioning considerations as presented in outline form on each positioning page. Learn the anatomy best demonstrated, the technical factors, the specific positioning steps, and the evaluation criteria for each projection or position.

Audio-visuals if available: Complete the audio-visual presentation for Part II if available before doing the review exercises in Part II of the workbook. Again do *not* write in the workbook during the audio-visual presentation.

Step 4. **Workbook and Laboratory Manual:** Complete the review exercises under Part II, Radiographic Positioning. As before, complete as many of the questions as you can before looking up the answers in the textbook or checking the answers on the answer sheet. You should then review the corresponding pages in the textbook again and repeat the audio-visuals if you missed more than the suggested minimum.

Step 5. **Workbook and Laboratory Manual (Laboratory Activity):** These exercises must be done in a radiographic laboratory using a phantom or a student model (without making exposure) with an energized radiographic unit and illuminators for viewing radiographs. Arrange for a time when you can use your radiographic lab or a diagnostic radiographic room in a clinic setting.

This is one of the most important aspects of this learning series and should not be neglected or de-emphasized. Experience has shown that students frequently have difficulty in transferring the information they have learned on positioning to actually positioning and correctly aligning a patient in a clinical setting. Therefore it is important that you carry out the laboratory activities as described in each chapter. Your instructors should assist you as needed in these exercises.

Anatomy Review: From radiographs provided by your instructor, review the anatomy by identifying each anatomical part as labeled on drawings and radiographs and described in your textbook and/or audio-visuals.

Film Critique: Critique and evaluate each radiograph for errors of less than optimal positioning or exposure factors based on evaluation criteria provided in the textbook and/or audiovisuals. Also, with the help of your instructor, begin to learn how to discriminate between those less than optimal, but passable radiographs, and those which need to be repeated. This generally requires additional experience and practice to be able to make such final judgements totally on your own without assistance from a supervising technologist or radiologist.

Self-Test

You should take the self-test only after you have completed the following:

1. Learning exercises, Part I Anatomy and Part II Positioning.

2. All laboratory activities.

3. Any supplementary reading as listed under Recommended Supplementary References.

4. Reviewed and checked off the objectives for this unit.

Take the self-test as in a regular test situation. After you have completed this test, check your answers with the answer sheet at the end of the chapter. If your score is less than 80%, you should go back and review the textbook and/or audio-visuals again paying special attention to the areas you missed.

Note: Even though 80% is given as the minimum passing achievement, any score less than 90% indicates that you really haven't mastered this material.

Chapter 1
Terminology and Principles
General Anatomy, Terminology, Imaging Principles, Radiation Protection, and Positioning Principles

Rationale

A major portion of the tasks of a Radiologic Technologist is centered around radiographic positioning. Therefore as a student in Radiologic Technology, it is imperative that you have a good understanding of anatomy, terminology, general imaging principles, radiation protection, and positioning principles.

This chapter is designed to introduce you to these important areas of medical radiographic positioning. The technical terminology used nationally to describe the various projections and views in radiographic positioning is important because you will soon be using them as part of your "everyday" language in Radiology. You also need to learn the correct pronunciation of these terms so you will become comfortable in using them. Hearing them pronounced correctly by the narrator in the audio-visuals will help you achieve this, as well as the phonetic respelling which is included for each new term in the textbook.

Understanding at least the basic imaging and radiation protection principles as described in this chapter is important as a foundation for all radiographic positioning.

Even though each anatomical part of the human body has its own "basic projections" or "routines," there are some general principles common in all positioning, which if understood will aid in learning the "basic projections" or "routines" for all anatomical parts. Learning and understanding these principles will help you develop a general understanding of positioning so you will not memorize specific routines for each body part. Instead you will understand why certain basic projections are taken and why modifications to these specific projections may be needed.

Chapter Objectives

After you have successfully completed **all** the activities of this chapter, you will be able, with at least 80% accuracy to:

___ 1. Understand the general anatomy and structural organization of the human body so that you will be able to describe the basic components at the chemical level of the body and list the four basic tissue types.

___ 2. List the ten body systems and describe specific functions of each.

___ 3. Identify the two parts or divisions of the skeletal system and identify the total number of bones in the average adult human body.

___ 4. Describe the primary and secondary bone formation centers.

___ 5. List the three primary **structural classifications** and the three **functional classifications** of joints, and list the six **movement types** with examples of each.

___ 6. Write a brief one sentence definition for each positioning term as described in the textbook and/or audio-visuals.

___ 7. When given an oral exam by an instructor, will be able to **orally describe** and/or **demonstrate** on yourself or another student each body position and body movement described in the textbook and/or audio-visuals.

___ 8. **Correctly** define the following terms: **positions, projections, and views.**

___ 9. List, define, and give controlling factors for the four image quality factors described in this chapter.

___ 10. Describe the ALARA principle of radiation protection and list specific ways this can be achieved for both the radiographer and the patient.

___ 11. Describe the two ways in which maximum collimation reduces patient dosage.

___ 12. Describe the ten-day rule, employed as a radiation protection practice.

___ 13. Describe the general positioning steps using both floating table top and fixed table top equipment.

___ 14. Write a short, accurate description of the two general principles or rules used in radiographic positioning as described in this chapter.

___ 15. List three reasons why most radiographic examinations require a **minimum** of two projections, 90° from each other.

___ 16. Discriminate between those radiographic examinations of the limbs requiring three projections and those requiring only two.

___ 17. Describe why examinations including joints in the primary interest area generally require three projections.

___ 18. List the three projections or positions which are required for examinations involving joints in the primary interest area.

Prerequisite

The reading level and the level of understanding needed to master this material is approximately that of a high school graduate. The flexibility of this learning method allows students of varying backgrounds to learn equally effectively. Students who have had previous courses in anatomy and physiology will probably be able to go through this course a little faster than those who have not, but the features of self-pacing and repetition allow all students the advantage of using this workbook and the associated textbook and/or audio-visuals equally effectively.

This first chapter is basic and does not use any terms which have not been previously defined. Therefore there is no prerequisite for this chapter.

Recommended Supplementary References

The recommended supplementary references are listed to provide the students with additional resources if they want more information on the material covered in this chapter. Even though all the information needed to meet the objectives of this chapter is provided in the Bontrager Textbook and/or the audio-visuals, it is suggested that at least one or two of the following references be read and studied for a more thorough understanding of this material. These references are listed in a suggested order of importance and value to understanding this information.

1. Merrill, V/Ballinger PW (ed). *Merrill's Atlas of Radiographic Positions and Radiologic Procedures*, 7th ed. St. Louis, MO. Mosby-Year Book, Inc.; 1991, Vol 1, pp 2-50

2. Swallow RA, Naylor E (ed). *Clark's Positioning in Radiography*, 11th ed. Rockville, MD. Aspen Publishing, Inc.; 1986, pp 2-31

3. Eisenberg RL, Dennis CA, May CR. *Radiographic Positioning*, Boston, MA. Little, Brown and Co.: 1989, pp 1-17

4. Bushong SC. *Radiologic Science for Technologists*, 4th ed. St. Louis, MO. Mosby-Year Book, Inc.; 1988, pp 290-307, 535-553

Learning Exercises

The following review exercises should be completed only after careful study of the associated pages in the textbook and/or audio-visuals as indicated by each exercise.

After completing each of these individual exercises, check your answers with the answers provided at the end of the review exercises.

Part I. GENERAL, SYSTEMIC AND SKELETAL ANATOMY AND ARTHROLOGY

Review Exercise A   Textbook: pp 1-13
                           Audio-visuals (Arthrology): Unit 6, slides 1-12

1. The lowest level of the structural organization of the human body is the chemical level wherein atoms are joined to form (a) _molecule_, which are organized to form (b) _cells_, which are the basic and structural unit of the entire body.
tissues - organs - systems

2. The four basic types of tissues of the body are: MENC

   A. _epithelicl_   C. _muscular_

   B. _connective_   D. _nervous_

3. The human body is made up of ten body systems which are:

   (1) _respiratory_   (6) _nervous_

   (2) _reproductive_   (7) _urinary_

   (3) _circulatory_   (8) _digestive_

   (4) _skeletal_   (9) _integumentary_

   (5) _muscular_   (10) _ENDOCRINE_

4. The average adult skeletal system consists of _208 (206)_ individual bones which are classified according to shape as a long bone, short bone, flat bone or irregular bone.

5. Red blood cells are produced by the red bone marrow of certain flat and irregular bones. Name two such bones.

   A. _ribs_   STERNUM

                   PELVIS

   B. _vertebra_

6. The first or primary center of bone formation (ossification) occurs in which area of the bone?

   the shaft   MIDSHAFT- DIAPHYSIS

7. The secondary centers of ossification wherein bone growth primarily occurs are called the

   (a) _*epiphysis*_ , which are separated from the primary bone by a space called the

   (b) _*epiphyseal plate*_ .

8. The study of joints or articulations is called _*arthrology*_ .

9. List the three primary **structural classifications** of joints (based on the type of tissue separating the ends of bone).

   A. _*synovial*_

   B. _*cartilagenous*_

   C. _*fibrous*_

10. The following joints would be classified in which of the above three classifications:

    A. Skull sutures _*fibrous*_

    B. Distal tibiofibular joint _*cartilagenous FIBROUS*_

    C. Symphysis pubis _*fibrous CARTILAGENOUS*_

    D. Intercarpal joints _*synovial*_

    E. Intervertebral discs _*synovial CARTILAGENOUS*_

    F. Knee joint _*synovial*_

11. The three **functional classifications** of joints based on their mobility or lack of mobility are:

    A. _*synarthrosis — no movement*_

    B. _*amphiarthrosis — some movement*_

    C. _*diarthrosis — freely moving*_

12. Freely movable joints are also classified by their **movement type** such as (1) gliding, (2) hinge, (3) pivot, (4) condyloid, (5) saddle and (6) ball and socket. Identify the movement type for the following joints. (Hint—all six movement types are included.)

    A. Hip joint _*ball & socket*_   E. Interphalangeal joints _*hinge*_

    B. Wrist joint _*gliding CONDYLOID*_   F. First carpometacarpal of thumb _*saddle*_

    C. Proximal and distal radioulnar joints _*pivot*_

    D. Intercarpal joints _*condyloid GLIDING*_
    *of wrist*

Part II. RADIOGRAPHIC TERMINOLOGY

Review Exercise B   General Terms, Projections and Positions

Textbook: pp 14-20
Audio-visuals: Unit 1, slides 1-26

Fill in definitions to the following terms. Use short precise answers.

1. X-ray film _the film before a picture is taken_
2. Radiograph _x-ray film with a picture on it_
3. Anatomical position _face forward, arms down, palms forward_
4. Supine (a) _lying face up_

   vs.

   Prone (b) _lying face down_
5. Posterior (a) _toward the back   DORSAL_

   vs.

   Anterior (b) _toward the front   VENTRAL_
6. PA (a) _posterioanterior   from back to front_

   vs.

   AP (b) _anterioposterior   from front to back_
7. Right lateral _right side closest to film_
8. RAO _right anterior oblique -rotated w/ rt ant. closest_
9. RPO _right posterior oblique -rotated w/rt. post closest_
10. Decubitus _lying down -(horizontal) ray_
11. Dorsal decub. (L lat.) _lying down -horizontal ray-on back -left closest_
12. R Lat. decub. (PA) _lying down-horizontal ray -on right side - back to front_
13. Recumbent _lying down ~~head higher than feet~~ any position_
14. Trendelenburg _lying down feet higher than head_
15. Ventral decub. (R lat.) _lying down -horizontal ray - face down- PRONE right close to film_
16. A true lateral chest would be rotated _90_ degrees from a true PA or AP.   OBLIQUE 45° to fil
17. Tangential _just touching an area -glancing_
18. Axial _along the long axis of the body_
19. Lordotic _swaybacked - shoulders on board, bent outward demonstrates apicies of lungs_

20. List the correct positioning terms for the following:
   A. Lying face-down on x-ray table, x-ray tube above, film below _prone PA_
   B. Lying on right side on x-ray table, x-ray tube above, film below _prone, rt lat recumbent_
   C. Standing, right anterior body surface placed against film _rt lat   RAO m. anterior oblique_
   D. Lying on x-ray table on left posterior body surface _LPO_
   E. Lying on right side, film in front of patient, x-ray tube behind _decubitus, rt lat PA_

Review Exercise C   Relationship Terms, Body Planes and Sections, Surfaces of Limbs
and Terms Related to Movements

Textbook: pp 21-28
Audio-visuals: Unit 1, slides 27-35

Fill in definitions to the following terms:

1. Cephalic _toward the head_
   vs.
2. Caudal _toward the feet (away from the head)_

3. Lateral _away from the midline_
   vs.
4. Medial _toward the midline_

5. Proximal _toward the trunk (source)_
   vs.
6. Distal _away from the trunk (source)_

7. Ipsilateral _on the same side_
   vs.
8. Contralateral _on opposite sides_

9. Plantar _bottom of foot_
   vs.
10. Dorsum (dorsum pedis) _top of foot_

11. Palmar (volar) _palm of the hand_

12. Flexion _bent - decreasing angle_
   vs.
13. Extension _straightened - increased angle_

14. Hyperextension _straighted beyond normal_

15. Eversion _turned outward (foot) STRESSED_
   vs.
16. Inversion _turned inward (foot) STRESSED_

17. Abduction ___away from body___

     vs.

18. Adduction ___toward body___

19. Supination ___hand palm upward___   lying face upward

     vs.

20. Pronation ___hand palm downward___   lying face downward

21. Protraction ___thrust outward (forward)___   jaw

     vs.

22. Retraction ___pulled inward (backward)___   jaw

23. Tilt ___turn off axis___

     vs.

24. Rotation ___turning on axis___

25. Midsagittal (median) plane ___cuts into 2 halves (left - right)___

26. A movement in which the angle of the joint is decreased: ___flexion___

27. An AP projection of the foot can also be described as a ___dorsiplantar___ projection.

28. A plantodorsal projection of the foot could also be described as a ___PA___ projection.

29. Are the fingers located **distal** or **proximal** to the wrist? ___distal___

30. The shoulder is **distal** or **proximal** to the elbow? ___proximal___

31. Fill in the correct term for the following movements:

     A. Movement of elbow joint as you touch your forehead: ___flexion___

     B. Movement of fingers as you close your hand: ___flexion___

     C. Moving your elbow laterally away from your body: ___abduction___

     D. Turning your palm up: (a) ___supination___; or down: (b) ___pronation___

     E. Moving your head back to look straight up at the sky: ___~~tilt~~ EXTENSION___

     F. Movement of your spine as you bend down to tie your shoe: ___flexion___

     G. Moving your arm down to your side from a raised position: ___adduction___

     H. Movement of foot as you raise up to a "tip-toe" position: ___~~plantar flexion~~ EXTENSION ANKLE___

     I. An inward "stress" movement of the foot: ___inversion___

32. The plane dividing the body into cephalic and caudal portions: ___transverse___

33. The plane dividing the body into unequal right and left portions: ___sagittal___   midsagittal (equal)

34. The plane dividing the body into anterior and posterior sections: ___coronal___

           MIDCORONAL

Part III. IMAGING PRINCIPLES

Review Exercise D   Image Quality Factors Textbook: pp 32-37

contrast = kVp variations

1. Define radiographic density. *amt of blackness*

2. The primary controlling factor for density is *mAs* _____.

3. The density change rule states that mAs must be changed at least (a) *30* % to make noticeable change, and increased at least (b) *50 100 DOUBLE* % to correct an underexposed radiograph.

4. Define radiographic contrast. *difference in density   variations*

5. The primary controlling factor for contrast is *kVp* _____.

6. A *15* % decrease in kVp generally is similar to cutting the mAs in half.   *15% Increase KVp = double mAs*

7. Low kVp results in (low or high) (a) *high* contrast, which is (short or long) (b) *short less variation* scale contrast.   *greater black/white variation*   *high kVp = low contrast = long scale contrast*

8. Recorded detail or definition can be defined as *sharpness of detail* *shades of gray* *structure on radiographic image*

9. The primary factor controlling or influencing detail is (a) *motion* _____. Additional controlling or influencing factors are (b) *SID* _____, (c) *OID* _____, and (d) *focal spot size* _____.

10. Identify one cause of loss of detail due to involuntary motion. *peristaltic movement* *heartbeat*

11. Define radiographic distortion. *diff in size or shape from reality*

12. The four primary controlling factors of distortion are (a) *SID* _____, (b) *OID* _____ (c) *alignment* _____ and (d) *central ray* _____, *CR*

13. Write in **increase** or **decrease** in each of these blanks. An increase in SID will (a) *decrease* distortion, will (b) *increase* recorded detail and will (c) *decrease* patient exposure.

14. Describe why there is **always** some magnification or distortion on any radiographic image. *because of the spreading of the ray* *DIVERGENCE*

15. Due to the anode heel effect, the intensity of the x-ray beam at the cathode end is **greater** or **lesser** than at the anode end. *greater*

16. The anode heel effect is greater with: (a) **smaller** or **larger** focal spot? *larger* *SMALLER*, (b) **smaller** or **larger** film? *larger*, and (c) **longer** or **shorter** SID? *shorter*

Part IV. PRINCIPLES OF RADIATION PROTECTION

Review Exercise E   Textbook: pp 38-42

1. The <u>MPD</u> (maximum permissible dose) for radiographers is (a) ___5___ rem per year and for the general public is (b) ___.5___ rem per year.

2. A more important protection principle is called ALARA. The initials stand for ___as low as___ ___reasonably achievable___

3. Name at least seven ways the ALARA principle can be achieved for both radiographers and patients.

   A. ___filtration___

   B. ___collimation___

   C. ___protection___ ___(shielding)___

   D. ___high kVp - optimum exposure factors___

   E. ___minimum repeat radiographs___

   F. ___always wear lead aprons___

   G. ___film badge___

4. Describe two ways which optimal collimation, to include only the area of interest, reduces patient exposure.

   A. ___other areas aren't unnecessarily exposed___

   B. ___less scatter radiation___

5. Describe the ten-day rule which ideally should be used for protection for pregnancies:

   ___x-rays should be taken in the first 10 days___ ___after onset of menstruation when there's the least___ ___chance of pregnancy___

Part V. BASIC PRINCIPLES OF RADIOGRAPHIC POSITIONING

Review Exercise F   Textbook: pp 43-48
Audio-visuals: Unit 1, slides 36-50

1. Describe the three general positioning steps using floating table top equipment wherein the part is positioned to the CR.

    A. _position the patient--with table locked_

    B. _position the film in the Bucky tray position CR to table & film_

    C. _position the CR unlock table to position correctly_

2. Describe the first general principle or rule in diagnostic radiology for determining positioning routines or the number of projections required. (A KUB abdomen is an exception.)

    two positions 90° from each other

3. Name three reasons for this general rule.

    A. _organs may be in the way ANATOMICAL STRUCTURES SUPERIMPOSED_

    B. _more than one necessary for exact identification LOCALIZATION OF LESIONS/ FOREIGN BODIES_

    C. _determine alignment of fractures DETERMINATION OF ALIGNMENT OF FRACTURES_

4. Describe a second positioning rule or principle related to the number of projections required for certain exams involving (joints.) _3 projections - because of many angles/surfaces involved_

5. Place an x under the basic projections required for each of the following:

    toes -3   hand -3
    knee -3   grip -2

	AP or PA	Lateral	Oblique
A. Ankle 3	X	X	X
B. Femur 2	X	X	
C. Chest 2	X	X	
D. Elbow 3	X	X	X
E. Fingers 3	X	X	X
F. Forearm 2	X	X	
G. Wrist 3	X	X	X
H. Foot 3	X	X	X
I. Leg (tibia-fibula) 2	X	X	~~X~~ NO
J. Foreign body in arm 2	X	X	

Review Exercise G   Laboratory Activity   Textbook: pp 16-29
                                                     Audio-visuals: Unit 1, slides 1-35

This learning activity exercise should be carried out in the radiographic laboratory or in a room or area where you can practice the various positioning terms described in this chapter.

You should now practice positioning the following positions and demonstrate the specific body movements on either yourself or another person. You should practice each of these until you can do them without hesitation. Place a check by each of the following as you achieve this.

___   1. Anatomical position

      2. Position a PA and AP of each of the following: (Use a pretend film and a table if you are not using the x-ray lab.)

___   a. Chest

___   b. Abdomen

___   c. Hand and forearm

___   d. Foot

___   e. Leg and knee

___   3. Position a right and left lateral of chest and abdomen.

      4. Position a chest and abdomen for the following obliques:

___   a. RAO

___   b. RPO

___   c. LPO

___   d. LAO

      5. Position a chest or abdomen for the following:

___   a. Right lateral decubitus

___   b. Left lateral decubitus

___   c. Dorsal decubitus

___   d. Ventral decubitus

      6. Practice demonstrations of the following specific body movements:

___   a. Flexion and extension of fingers, wrist, and elbow

___   b. Flexion and extension of foot and knee

___   c. Flexion and extension of spine including neck

___   d. Abduction of arm and leg

___   e. Adduction of arm and leg

___   f. Pronation and supination of hand and arm

Answers to Review Exercise A

1. (a) molecules   (b) cells

2. A. Epithelial
   B. Connective
   C. Muscular
   D. Nervous

3. (1) Skeletal
   (2) Circulatory
   (3) Digestive
   (4) Respiratory
   (5) Urinary
   (6) Reproductive
   (7) Nervous
   (8) Muscular
   (9) Endocrine
   (10) Integumentary

4. 206

5. A. Sternum
   B. Ribs
       (Other possible answers: vertebrae or pelvis)

6. Midshaft area or diaphysis

7. A. Epiphysis
   B. Epiphyseal plates

8. Arthrology

9. A. Fibrous joints
   B. Cartilaginous joints
   C. Synovial joints

10. A. Fibrous
    B. Fibrous
    C. Cartilaginous
    D. Synovial
    E. Cartilaginous
    F. Synovial

11. A. Synarthrosis (immovable)
    B. Amphiarthrosis (limited movement)
    C. Diarthrosis (freely movable)

12. A. Ball and socket
    B. Condyloid
    C. Pivot
    D. Gliding
    E. Hinge
    F. Saddle

If you missed more than 8 blanks, you should review this section again in the textbook and/or audio-visuals before continuing to the next section.

Answers to Review Exercise B

1. The film used in radiology before it has been exposed and processed.

2. The x-ray film after it has been exposed and processed, and contains an image.

3. An upright position with the arms down (adducted at sides), palms forward, and the head facing forward anteriorly.

4. (a) A patient lying on his or her back.
   (b) A patient lying on his or her abdomen.

5. (a) The back or dorsal surface.
   (b) The front or ventral surface.

6. (a) X-ray beam enters at posterior surface and exits at anterior.
   (b) X-ray beam enters at anterior and exits at posterior surface.

7. The patient's right side against the film (rotated ninety degrees from a true AP or PA).

8. Right anterior oblique (patient rotated with right anterior or front closest to the film).

9. Right posterior oblique (patient rotated with right posterior or back surface closest to the film).

10. The patient lying down in any position using a horizontal x-ray beam.

11. Lying on back, using horizontal beam, left side against film.

12. Lying on right side, using horizontal beam, anterior surface against film.

13. Lying down in any position.

14. Recumbent position with body plane tilted so head is lower than feet.

15. Lying on abdomen, using horizontal beam, right side against film.

16. 90

17. A projection which skims a body part projecting it away from other body structures.

18. The long axis of the body or part around which a body or part rotates (also used to indicate any angle of the x-ray beam along the long axis of the body).

19. A descriptive term for a special chest projection demonstrating the apices of the lungs.

20. A. Prone position, PA projection
    B. Right lateral position
    C. Right anterior oblique or RAO
    D. Left posterior oblique or LPO
    E. Right lateral decub. (PA)

If you missed more than 5 blanks, you should review this section again in the textbook and/or audio-visuals before continuing to the next section.

Answers to Review Exercise C

1. Toward head

2. Toward feet

3. Away from center or midline

4. Toward the center or midline

5. Near the source or beginning of structure

6. Away from the source or beginning of structure

7. On the same side of body or part

8. On the opposite side of body or part

9. Sole or posterior surface of foot

10. Top or anterior surface of foot

11. The palm of hand

12. Flexing or bending joint, angle of joint is decreased

13. Straightening joint or increasing angle of joint

14. Extending joint beyond the straight or neutral position

15. Outward stress movement of foot

16. Inward stress movement of foot

17. Movement away from body

18. Movement toward body

19. Movement of the body, or an anatomical part, toward a supine position.

20. Movement of the body, or an anatomical part, toward a prone position.

21. A forward movement from normal position

22. A backward movement from normal position

23. A slanting or tilting movement with respect to the long axis

24. A rotation or turning of a body part on its axis

25. Plane dividing body into right and left halves (equal parts)

26. Flexion

27. Dorsoplantar

28. PA

29. Distal

30. Proximal

31. A. Flexion
    B. Flexion
    C. Abduction
    D. (a) supination (b) pronation
    E. Extension
    F. Flexion
    G. Adduction
    H. Extension
    I. Inversion

32. Transverse

33. Sagittal

34. Coronal

If you missed more than 6 blanks, you should review this section again in the textbook and/or audio-visuals before continuing to the next section.

Answers to Review Exercise D

1. The degree or amount of blackening on a radiograph.

2. mAs

3. (a) 30 (b) 100

4. The difference in density on adjacent areas of a radiographic image.

5. kVp

6. 15

7. (a) High
   (b) Short

8. The sharpness of structures on a radiographic image

9. (a) Motion
   (b) Focal spot size
   (c) SID (source image receptor distance)
   (d) OID (object image receptor distance)

10. Peristaltic action of abdominal organs

11. Misrepresentation of object size or shape recorded on a radiographic image

12. (a) SID
    (b) OID
    (c) Object alignment
    (d) CR (central ray) location

13. (a) decrease
    (b) increase
    (c) decrease

14. Because of the divergence of the x-ray beam from a point source in the x-ray tube.

15. Greater

16. (a) Smaller
    (b) Larger
    (c) Shorter

If you missed more than 6 blanks, you should review this section again in the textbook and/or audio-visuals before continuing to the next section.

Answers to Review Exercise E

1. (a) 5 (b) .5

2. "As Low As Reasonably Achievable"

3. a. Radiographers always wear a film badge.
   b. Persons restraining patients (never radiology personnel) always wear lead apron and gloves and stay out of primary beam.
   c. Radiographers doing portables, trauma exams, or fluoroscopy always wear lead apron and gloves
   d. Do minimum repeat radiographs
   e. Use correct filtration
   f. Always use accurate collimation
   g. Use specific area (gonadal) shielding for all patients of child bearing age or younger
      Additional correct answers:
      Use maximum protection for pregnancies, or
      Use optimum exposure factors and high speed screen-film combinations

4. A. Reducing the volume of tissue directly irradiated
   B. Reducing the accompanying scatter radiation which also exposes patients

5. All radiologic examinations involving the female pelvis or lower abdomen should be scheduled during the first ten days following the onset of menstruation.

If you missed more than 3 blanks, you should review this section again in the textbook and/or audio-visuals before continuing to the next section.

Answers to Review Exercise F

1. A. Patient is placed on table into correct body position with table in a locked position.
   B. CR is aligned and centered to film at correct SID and angling of CR if required.
   C. Table-top is unlocked and patient and table-top are moved as needed to align the CR to the correct centering point on patient.

2. A minimum of two projections should be taken as near 90° from each other as possible for most exams.

3. A. Certain conditions may not be visible on one projection due to superimposition of other structures.
   B. Necessary for localization of lesions or foreign bodies.
   C. Necessary for determination of alignment of fractures.

4. Radiographic exams including joints in the primary interest area require three projections, an AP or PA, a lateral and an oblique.

5.

	AP or PA	Lateral	Oblique
A.	x	x	x
B.	x	x	
C.	x	x	
D.	x	x	x
E.	x	x	x
F.	x	x	
G.	x	x	x
H.	x	x	x
I.	x	x	
J.	x	x	

If you missed more than 7 blanks, you should review this section again in the textbook and/or audio-visuals before continuing.

Self-Test

My score = _____ %

Directions: After you have completed all of the learning activity exercises including the laboratory activities and think each chapter objective has been achieved, then take this self-test.

Scoring will not affect your grade. For this to have any value for you, you should simulate actual test conditions when completing this self-test. This is your opportunity to identify those tasks which you have mastered as well as possible deficiencies.

After you have completed this task, check your answers with the answer sheet which follows this test.

For calculating your percentage grade, use the number of points per question, as indicated below. If your score is over 80%, you may continue to the final chapter evaluation. A score of less than 80% indicates that you should go back and review the associated pages in the textbook and/or audio-visuals, the review exercises in the workbook, and pay special attention to the areas you missed on this test.

Even though a score of 80% is used to indicate success, a score of less than 90% really indicates that you haven't truly mastered the material and it would be beneficial for you to review your weak areas before taking the final chapter evaluation provided by your instructor. Good luck!

Test

There are 100 blanks. Each correct answer is worth 1 point.

Complete the following by filling in the term(s) which best describe(s) each of the following. (Spelling is important so correct any misspellings as you grade your test.)

1. Patient lying flat on his/her back on stretcher _____supine_____

2. Patient lying on right side on x-ray table (tube overhead and film under patient) _R lat. recumbent_

3. Patient facing the chest film with x-ray tube behind, turned slightly, with right shoulder against film
   _RAO PA_____

4. Patient lying on abdomen, face down on stretcher _prone_____

5. Patient lying on the x-ray table, turned up slightly on right posterior hip _RPO_____

6. Patient standing with back flat against the chest film with x-ray tube in front _AP_____

7. Same as #6 but turned slightly toward patient's right _AP   RPO_____

8. Patient lying directly on left side, x-ray tube above and film under _L lat recumbent_____

9. The correct term for an x-ray film after it has been exposed, processed, and contains an anatomical image _radiograph_

10. The correct term which describes a person standing, arms at sides, palms forward, feet and head directed forward or anterior _anatomical position_

11. An inward "stress" movement of the foot as it remains in an AP position _inversion_

12. The term used most commonly to refer to the back of a patient _posterior_   DORSAL

13. Is the top of the foot the **anterior** or **posterior** surface? _anterior_   VENTRAL

14. The term describing the position of the hand when it is rotated 45° from a PA or AP _lateral_ OBL

15. Patient lying face down on x-ray table but turned up slightly on left shoulder and hip _prone_ RAO

16. The position a patient would be in if turned exactly half-way between a PA and a right lateral position _oblique_   RAO

17. Patient lying on right side on stretcher with the film behind and the x-ray tube in front (using horizontal beam) _Rt lat decubitus (AP)_

18. The term referring to an angle away from the head end of the patient _tangential_ CAUDAL

19. The term most commonly used in referring to the palm of the hand _palmar_ (VOLAR)

20. The wrist is located _distal_ to the elbow.

21. A dorsoplantar projection of the foot could also be described as a _AP_ projection.

22. The movement of your spine as you bend down to tie your shoe _flexion_

23. The term describing the lateral movement of your arm away from your body _abduction_

24. The movement of your elbow joint as you bring your arm up from your side and touch your head _flexion_

25. The movement whereby the angle of a joint is decreased _flexion_

26. The rotation of your hand so the palm is facing up _supination_

27. The movement of your spine as you look up directly at the sky _extension_

28. The plane dividing the body into left and right halves _midsagittal_   sagittal 2 unequal pa

29. The movement whereby the degree of angle of a joint is increased _extension_

30. A term referring to parts away from the head end of the body _distal_ CAUDAL
distal - away from the trunk

31. A second term other than anterior used to refer to the top of the foot _dorsal_ DORSUM PEDIS

32. The rotation of your hand so the palm is facing down ___pronation___

33. A plane dividing the body into anterior and posterior portions ___coronal___

34. Angle of the x-ray beam toward the head ___cranial   CEPHALIC___

35. The patient lying on back with the film against right side and the x-ray tube on left side using a horizontal beam ___supine DORSAL decubitus rt.___

36. Movement of your foot as you move your toes down as far as possible ___plantar flexion___ EXTENSION OF ANKLE

37. A specific term referring to the sole or posterior surface of the foot ___plantar___

38. Patient lying on left side on a stretcher facing the x-ray table with the x-ray tube behind (using horizontal beam) ___decubitus left lat PA___

39. The body plane dividing the body into cephalic and caudal portions ___transverse___

40. The four basic types of tissues, which when connected together, perform specific functions:

    A. ___connective___   C. ___muscular___

    B. ___epithelial___   D. ___nervous___

41. The human body is made up of ten body systems each performing specific functions. Identify the body system which performs the following functions:

    A. Produces blood cells and stores calcium. ___skeletal___ sternum, ribs pelvis, vertebra

    B. Transports water, electrolytes, hormones, and enzymes, and helps to regulate body temperatures.

    ___circulatory___

    C. Reproduces the organism. ___reproductive___

    D. Supplies oxygen to the blood and to body cells, and assists in regulating the acid-base balance of the blood. ___respiratory___

    E. Regulates the chemical composition of the blood, and eliminates many waste products.

    ___urinary___

    F. Regulates body activities through various hormones carried by the cardiovascular system.

    ___endocrine___

    G. Allows for movements of the body, and produces heat. ___muscular___

    H. Protects the body, and eliminates waste products through perspiration. ___integumentary___

42. The total number of bones in an average adult is ___206___.

respiratory
reproductive
endocrine
integumentary
skeletal

muscular
circulatory
nervous
digestive
urinary

43. All bones of the body can be classified according to shape into four types or classes. A. _long_
    B. _short_   C. _flat_   D. _irregular_

44. Red blood cells are produced in two of these classifications of bones . Which are they?
    A. _flat_   B. _irregular_

45. Each **secondary** center of ossification or bone formation wherein growth occurs is called an
    epiphysis.

46. The **primary** center of ossification in long bones occurs in the **midshaft** area which is called the
    diaphysis.

47. The three **structural** classifications of joints are:
    A. _synovial_
    B. _cartilagenous_
    C. _FIBROUS_

48. Which of the above classifications allows the most movements?
    synovial

49. What terms describe the following mobility classifications:
    A. Freely movable? _DIARTHROTIC_ ~~amphiarthrotic~~
    B. Immovable? _synarthrotic_
    C. Slightly movable? _AMPHIARTHROTIC_ ~~diarthrotic~~

50. Which two types of markers should be used on every radiograph. (A radiograph taken without these two
    markers generally should be repeated.)
    A. _left or right_
    B. _position PATIENT ID WITH DATE_

51. List the **primary** controlling or influencing factor(s) for each of the following:
    A. Contrast _— kVp_
    B. Density _— mAs_
    C. Detail (definition) _~~mAs~~ MOTION   SID, OID, FOCAL SPOT SIZE_
    D. Distortion _~~movement~~ not proper A→E or shape, alignment, _SID_, and _OID_.

52. The best way to reduce or minimize image unsharpness caused by involuntary motion is _____
    reduce time of exposure.

53. High contrast is the result of _____low_____ kVp. (high or low)   *short → high contrast*   *black/white*

54. Long scale contrast is the result of _____high_____ kVp. (high or low)   *long → low contrast*   *grays*

55. A 15% increase in kVp will increase density about the same as a __100__ % increase in mAs.   *DOUBLE*

56. The purpose of contrast is _to define features -MAKE DETAIL MORE VISIBLE_.

57. True or false:

    _T_ A. Some magnification and/or distortion is **always** present on a radiograph.

    _F_ B. An increase in SID increases distortion.

    _T_ C. A decrease in OID decreases distortion.

    _F_ D. To minimize anode heel effect, the largest part of the patient should be placed at the anode end of the x-ray tube   *cathode - greater intensity*

    _T_ E. All general purpose x-ray machines are required by law to have automatic collimation devices which automatically collimate to the film size in the bucky tray.

    _F_ F. The film badge worn on the collar of the technologist should be under the lead apron during fluoroscopy to determine accurate body dose.

    _T_ G. An increase in SID and a decrease in OID will increase geometric sharpness or detail.

58. What two projections should always be taken when the body part is in a cast to aid the physician in determining alignment of fractures?

    A. _PA /AP_   *2 views 90° apart*

    B. _lateral_

59. List three reasons why at least two projections are generally taken as a basic routine for all or most radiographic exams:

    A. _anatomical superimposure_

    B. _location of lesions/ foreign objects_

    C. _alignment of fractures_

60. Which three projections are routinely taken when joints are in the prime interest area?

    A. _AP /PA_

    B. _lateral_

    C. _oblique_

61. Indicate the **minimum** number of projections which should routinely be taken for the following:

| A. Knee _3_ | C. Forearm _2_ | E. Chest _2_ | G. Humerus _2_ |
| B. Foot _3_ | D. Elbow _3_ | F. Fingers _3_ | H. Femur _2_ |

Answers to Self Test

1. Supine
2. Right lateral
3. RAO or right anterior oblique
4. Prone
5. RPO or right posterior oblique
6. AP or anteroposterior
7. RPO or right posterior oblique
8. Left lateral
9. Radiograph
10. Anatomical position
11. Inversion
12. Posterior
13. Anterior
14. Oblique
15. LAO or left anterior oblique
16. 45° RAO or right anterior oblique
17. Right lateral decubitus (AP)
18. Caudal
19. Palmar surface
20. Distally
21. AP or anteroposterior
22. Flexion
23. Abduction
24. Flexion
25. Flexion
26. Supination

27. Extension
28. Midsagittal
29. Extension
30. Caudal (inferior)
31. Dorsum pedis
32. Pronation
33. Coronal
34. Cephalic (superior)
35. Dorsal decubitus (R lat.)
36. Extension
37. Plantar
38. Left lateral decubitus (PA)
39. Transverse plane
40. A. Epithelial
    B. Connective
    C. Muscular
    D. Nervous
41. A. Skeletal system
    B. Circulatory system
    C. Reproductive system
    D. Respiratory system
    E. Urinary system
    F. Endocrine system
    G. Muscular system
    H. Integumentary system
42. 206
43. A. Long
    B. Short
    C. Flat
    D. Irregular
44. A. Flat
    B. Irregular
45. Epiphysis
46. Diaphysis

47. A. Fibrous joints
    B. Cartilaginous joints
    C. Synovial joints

48. Synovial

49. A. Diarthrodial
    B. Synarthrodial
    C. Amphiarthrodial

50. A. Patient identification including date
    B. Anatomical side marker

51. A. kVp
    B. mAs
    C. Motion
    D. SID, OID, object alignment, CR

52. A short exposure time

53. Low

54. High

55. 100

56. To make the detail of a radiograph more visible

57. A. True
    B. False
    C. True
    D. False
    E. True
    F. False
    G. True

58. A. AP or PA
    B. Lateral or 90° from the PA or AP

59. A. The problem of anatomical structures being
       superimposed on one projection only
    B. Necessary for localization of lesions or
       foreign bodies
    C. Necessary for determining alignment of fractures

60. A. AP or PA
    B. Oblique
    C. Lateral

61. A. 3   C. 2   E. 2   G. 2
    B. 3   D. 3   F. 3   H. 2

Chapter 2
Chest

Rationale

The most common of all radiographic examinations is that of the chest. This is probably the first type of radiographic examination that you will perform as students in Radiologic Technology.

Even though this is considered one of the easier examinations, in many departments chests are the most frequently repeated exam. The reason for this is probably related to the simplicity and routineness of this exam and the way chests have traditionally been positioned and centered using the relationship of the top of the film to the top of the shoulders as the centering method. This "shot gun" approach to chest centering causes students and technologists to develop careless habits which result in inaccurate positioning with resultant poor chest radiographs. When this happens, the radiologist interpreting the chest radiograph may misinterpret or even completely miss some important pathology present in the chest but not visible on the radiograph because of superimposition or distortion caused by inaccurate patient positioning.

It has been said that there is more potential pathology or more possible abnormal conditions or diseases present in the chest than any other part of the body. This obviously makes it important to be very accurate in both positioning and exposure factors when taking chest radiographs.

The purpose of this chapter is to help you learn and understand both the anatomy and positioning routines of the chest utilizing an accurate central ray to center the lung fields to the center of the cassette. This "rifle" approach to chest centering consistently centers the central ray to the center of the lung fields and provides for accurate collimation on patients of all types and sizes (body habitus).

You will learn how to view a chest radiograph to check for accuracy of positioning, centering, collimation and optimum exposure factors. When you start taking chest radiographs, you will be able to evaluate them using the evaluation criteria described in the textbook and/or audio-visuals to see if you are achieving the degree of accuracy for which you are striving.

Chapter Objectives

After you have successfully completed **all** the activities of this unit, you will be able, with at least 80% accuracy to: (applicable to a written and/or oral examination and demonstration)

___ 1. List and identify on drawings, the structures constituting the airway through which oxygen will pass as it travels from the nose and mouth to the terminal aspects of the lungs.

___ 2. Name and identify on drawings, the structure serving as a common passageway for both food and air.

___ 3. Identify the topographical landmarks used for locating the central ray on PA and AP chest radiographs and describe how the central point of the lungs is located on an average male and female patient utilizing these landmarks.

___ 4. List the skeletal landmarks associated with organs of the respiratory system as described in the textbook and/or audio-visuals.

___ 5. Identify on drawings and radiographs, the anatomical parts and relationships of the bony thorax, larynx, trachea, bronchi, lungs and mediastinal structures as identified in the textbook and/or audio-visuals.

___ 6. Identify which bronchus food particles (if aspirated) are most likely to enter, and explain why.

___ 7. List the number of ribs which should be demonstrated above the diaphragm on an optimum erect PA chest radiograph.

___ 8. Discriminate between PA and lateral chest radiographs with and without rotation.

___ 9. Describe three reasons for taking chest radiographs in the erect position whenever possible.

___10. Simulate taking AP, PA and lateral chest radiographs on a model posing as an ambulatory and a wheelchair patient.

___11. Take an AP supine chest radiograph on a full body phantom and produce a satisfactory radiograph **or** if this equipment is not available, simulate the same on a model without making an exposure.

Given several chest radiographs to view:

___12. Identify all visible anatomy of the lungs and thorax as described and illustrated in the textbook and/or audio-visuals.

___13. Critique and evaluate each radiograph based on evaluation criteria provided in the textbook and/or audio-visuals.

___14. Discriminate between radiographs which are acceptable and those which are unacceptable due to exposure factors, motion, collimation and/or positioning errors.

Prerequisite

The only prerequisite knowledge requirement for this chapter is an understanding of radiographic terminology and the principles of exposure, radiation protection, and positioning as described in Chapter 1. It is strongly suggested that a mandatory prerequisite for this chapter be the successful completion of Chapter 1.

Recommended Supplementary References

The recommended supplementary references are listed to provide you with additional resources if you want more information on the material covered in this chapter. Even though all the information needed to meet the objectives of this chapter is provided in the Bontrager Textbook and/or the audio-visuals, it is suggested that at least one or two of the following references be read and studied for a more thorough understanding of this material. The following references, which are described in more detail in Chapter 1, are listed in a suggested order of importance and value to understanding this material.

1. *Merrill's ...*, Vol. 2, pp 395-434

2. *Clark's ...*, pp 278-307

3. *Eisenberg ...*, pp 23-35

Learning Exercises

The following review exercises should be completed only after careful study of the associated pages in the textbook and/or the audio-visuals as indicated by each exercise.

After completing each of these individual exercises, check your answers with the answers provided at the end of the review exercises.

Part I RADIOGRAPHIC ANATOMY

Review Exercise A   Anatomy of the Larynx, Trachea, Bronchi, Lungs and Mediastinal Structures

> Textbook: pp 49-57
> Audio-visuals: Unit 2, slides 1-19

1. The bony thorax consists of the single (a) _sternum_ anteriorly, two (b) _clavicles_,
    two (c) _scapulas_ SCAPULAE, twelve pairs of (d) _ribs_ and twelve (e) _vertebra_ THORACIC
    posteriorly. _thorax - ribs, sternum, vertebra_
    shoulder girdle - clavicle, scapulas

2. An important bony landmark of the thorax used for locating the central ray on a PA chest is the
    ~~cartilage~~ VERTEBRA PROMINENS.

3. List the preferred name and the two secondary names for the bony landmark used for locating the central
    ray on an AP chest:
    A. Preferred name _JUGULAR NOTCH_
    B. Secondary names _~~adams apple~~ MANUBRIAL NOTCH_ or _SUPRASTERNAL NOTCH_

4. The four divisions of the respiratory system are:
    A. _~~trachea~~ LARYNX   voicebox_
    B. _phar~~ynx~~ TRACHEA_
    C. _bronchi_
    D. _lungs_

5. What is the correct anatomical term for the following:
    A. Adam's Apple _thyroid cartilage_   D. Shoulder blade _scapula_
    B. Voice box _larynx_   E. Collar bone _clavicle_
    C. Breastbone _sternum_

6. List the three divisions of the structure located proximally to the larynx which serves as a common
    passageway for both food and air?
    A. _nasopharynx_
    B. _~~oro~~pharynx_
    C. _LARYNGOPHARYNX_

7. What is the name of the structure which acts as a lid over the larynx to prevent foreign objects such as food particles from entering the respiratory system? _epiglottis_

8. Is the trachea located anteriorly or posteriorly to the esophagus? _anterior_

9. List the skeletal landmarks (specific vertebrae) identified with the following:

A. Upper margin of larynx _C3_

B. Lower margin of larynx _C6_

C. Thyroid cartilage (prominent portion) _C5_

D. Upper margin of trachea _C6_

E. Lower margin of trachea _T4 or T5_

10. The small bone in the anterior portion of the neck from which the larynx is suspended is the _hyoid_ bone.

11. If a person accidentally inhales a food particle, which bronchus is it most likely to enter and why?

A. _right_ bronchus

B. Why? _larger diameter, smaller angle (MORE VERTICAL)_

12. What is the name of the prominence or ridge as seen looking down into the bronchus where it divides into the right and left bronchi? _CARINA_   _T4-T5_

13. Identify which lung has three lobes and name each lobe.

A. _right_ lung

B. _upper_ , _middle_ , and _lower_ lobes.

14. What is the term defining the small air sacs located at the distal ends of the bronchioles where oxygen and carbon dioxide are exchanged in the blood? _alveoli_

15. A. The double-walled membrane containing the lungs is the _pleura_ .

B. The outer layer adhering to the inner surface of the chest wall is the _parietal pleura_

C. The inner layer adhering to the surface of the lungs is the _pulmonary_ or _visceral pleura_ .

D. The potential space between these two layers is the _pleural cavity_ , which when filled with air, can cause the lung to collapse, a condition called _pneumothorax_ .

16. Fill in the correct terms for the following portions of the lungs:

A. Broad lower portion _base_

B. Area where bronchi enter lungs _hilum_

C. Upper rounded portion above clavicles _apex (apices)_

pneumo - air in the pleural cavity

atelectasis - collapsed lung

17. Identify the term for the potential space or area in the thoracic cavity located between the lungs.

    mediastinum

18. List the four primary structures located in this space.

    A. *heart ↓ LARGE VESSELS*

    B. *large vessels   TRACHEA*

    C. *thymus gland*

    D. *esophagus*

19. Which lung is shorter or which hemidiaphragm is normally positioned higher and why?

    A. *right* lung or hemidiaphragm is higher.

    B. Why? *it has to make room for the liver*

20. What term describes the extreme lateral aspects or points where the diaphragm meets the ribs?

    costophrenic angle

21. List the structures through which air will pass as it travels from the nose and mouth to the alveoli of the lungs:

    A. Nose and mouth

    B. *pharynx*

    C. *larynx*

    D. *trachea*

    E. *bronchi*

    F. Alveoli of lungs

22. The heart is enclosed in a double-walled membrane or sac called the *pericardium* *PERICARDIAL SAC* .

23. Approximately two-thirds of the heart lies to the *left* (right or left) of the median plane.

PART II RADIOGRAPHIC POSITIONING

Review Exercise B   Technical and Positioning Considerations   Textbook: pp 58-77
                                                             Audio-visuals: Unit 2, slides 20-93

1. Fill in the correct term defining each of the following variations in the form and shape of the body (body habitus):

   A. Broad deep thorax? _HYPERSTHENIC_

   B. Long and slender thorax, narrow in width and shallow from front to back? _ASTHENIC_

   C. The two types making up the majority (85%) of the population are the _STHENIC (50%)_
   and _HYPOSTHENIC (35%)_.

2. What is the minimum number of ribs which should be demonstrated above the diaphragm on a good PA chest radiograph? _10_

3. Chest radiography generally is done with (low or high) (a) _low_ contrast, which requires (low or high) (b) _high_ kVp.

4. Describe the general rule or criterion for determining if there is sufficient density on a PA chest radiograph. _ribs +vertebrae are slightly visible through the heart_

5. List four possible conditions or pathologies which would suggest the need for both inspiration and expiration PA chest radiographs:

   A. _pneumothorax_

   B. _fluid in lungs_ LACK OF MOVEMENT OF DIAPHRAGM

   C. _FOREIGN BODY_

   D. _DISTINGUISH BETWEEN OPACITY OF RIB OR LUNG_

6. List the three reasons chest radiographs should be taken in an erect position if the patient's condition allows:

   A. _lower diaphragm_

   B. _prevent engorgement of pulmonary arteries_

   C. _SHOW POSSIBLE AIR + FLUID LEVELS_

7. Why should chest radiographs be taken at 72" SID? _to eliminate distortion of size of heart_   MINIMIZE MAGNIFICATION

8. Why will the lungs tend to expand more in an erect position than in a supine position? _other organs are out of the way_ DIAPHRAGM CAN MOVE DOWN FARTHER

9. Why is it especially important to take chest radiographs in an erect position when the patient's chart indicates possible fluid in the lungs? _so the fluid collects at the bottom of the lungs_

10. Describe two ways rotation can be determined on each of the following:

   A. PA chest radiograph _distance to ribs ^not equal_ and/or _sternoclavicular joint ^not equal distance from sternum_

   B. Lateral chest radiograph _diaphragms ^not superimposed_ and/or _ribs ^not superimposed at spine POSTERIOR RIBS OR COSTOPHRENIC ANGLES NOT SUPERIMPOSED_

11. Which lateral (right or left) position would you take for the following:

   A. Patient with severe pains in left chest _left_

   B. Patient with no chest pain but history of pneumonia in right lung _right_

   C. Patient has no chest pain and no history of heart trouble _left_

12. Why is it important to raise the patient's arms above his or her head on a lateral chest radiograph? _to keep flesh from arms away from lungs_

13. Which film marker should be used and where should it be placed on the film for the following:

   A. PA erect chest _L - top left_

   B. Left lateral chest _L - top right_

   C. Right lateral chest _R - top left_

14. The average height of lung fields is _less_ (greater or less) than the width.

15. Describe how to locate the central ray on the following:

   A. PA chest, average female _7" INFERIOR TO VERTEBRA PROMINENS_

   B. PA chest, average male _____

   C. PA chest, athletic, well developed male _____

   D. AP chest, average male or female _____

   E. AP chest, young athletic type _____

16. For a PA chest radiograph on a hypersthenic patient, should the 14 x 17" cassette be placed lengthwise or crosswise? _crosswise_

17. For a PA chest the top border of the light field (as shown on the back of the patient) should be adjusted to the level of the _VERTEBRA PROMINENS_ .

PA chest → cephalic

18. To prevent the clavicles from obscuring the apices of the lungs on an AP chest, the CR should be angled

slightly (a) ___CAUDAL___ so as to be perpendicular to the long axis of the (b) ___STERNUM___ .

19. Why should a 14 x 17" film holder be placed crosswise on all AP supine chests? _____

___because the person is laying down___ *TO PREVENT CUTOFF OF LUNG MARGINS DUE TO SMALLER SID*

20. Which lateral decubitus chest position (right or left lateral) should be taken for the following:

A. Possible **fluid** in pleural cavity of **left** lung? ___left___

B. Possible **air** in pleural cavity (pneumothorax) of **right** lung? ___left___

21. Which oblique chest position should be taken, and how much should the patient be rotated for a study of

the heart? ___left   LAO   60°___

22. What are the suggested basic projections/positions for a chest? ___PA, left lat.___

23. List three of the most common optional projections/positions taken for the chest in the U.S.

A. ___lordotic___   *AP SUPINE*

B. ___Oblique___

C. ___decub. lateral___

24. For a true lateral chest, the side away from the film generally needs to be rotated slightly (a) ___anteriorly___

(anteriorly or posteriorly). Why? (b) ___divergence of the ray___

Review Exercise C   Laboratory Activity   Textbook: pp 66-76

This part of the learning activity exercise series needs to be carried out in a radiographic laboratory or diagnostic room in a radiology department where facilities for chest radiography are available.

Positioning Exercise

For this section you need another person to act as your "patient" and you should go through **ALL** the steps (except making exposure) as outlined in the textbook and/or audio-visuals. Practice the following until you can do each of them accurately and without hesitation. Place a check by each when you have achieved this.

Include the following details as you simulate each of the following projections/positions:

- correct placement of film holder
- correct placement of marker
- correct patient positioning
- correct placement of lead shields
- correct CR location and collimation
- approximate correct exposure technique
- correct breathing instructions as you simulate the exposure

___ 1. PA chest: Include all steps from the time the ambulatory patient walks in the door until the exposure is "simulated." (May omit undressing and putting on a hospital gown.)

___ 2. Lateral chest following the PA projection.

___ 3. PA and lateral chest with patient in wheelchair. (Patient is too weak to stand.)

___ 4. AP, left lateral decubitus chest.

___ 5. AP supine chest on an "unconscious" patient.

___ 6. Anterior and posterior oblique chest positions.

___ 7. AP and a lateral upper airway.

Optional

___ 8. If a full-body phantom is available, take a supine chest to produce a satisfactory radiograph with correct positioning and correct technical factors including density, contrast, and film marker placement.

Review Exercise D Film Critique and Evaluation Textbook: pp 66-76

Your instructor will provide various chest radiographs for these exercises. These should include PA, lateral, obliques, lateral decubitus and AP lordotic projections, some of which should be well positioned radiographs with optimum exposure factors and correct patient ID and marker placement based on evaluation criteria provided for each projection in the textbook and/or audio-visuals. Several of these radiographs should be unacceptable requiring repeat exams and others should be less than optimal as to positioning, exposure factors, collimation errors and/or patient ID or marker placement.

Place a check by each of the following when it is completed.

___ 1. Examine several PA chest radiographs and count specific vertebra and ribs to determine correct CR location and the depth of inspiration on each PA projection.

___ 2. Critique each radiograph based on evaluation criteria provided for that projection in the textbook and/or audio-visuals. The following criteria guidelines can be used and checked as each radiograph is evaluated.

Radiographs						Criteria Guidelines
1	2	3	4	5	6	
—	—	—	—	—	—	a. Transverse (side to side) centering?
—	—	—	—	—	—	b. Lengthwise (top-to-bottom) centering?
—	—	—	—	—	—	c. Correct collimation?
—	—	—	—	—	—	d. Rotation?
—	—	—	—	—	—	e. Motion?
—	—	—	—	—	—	f. Exposure: density, and/or contrast?
—	—	—	—	—	—	g. Patient ID information and markers?

___ 3. Based on acceptable variances to criteria factors, determine which of these radiographs are acceptable and which are unacceptable and should have been repeated.

Important: It is important that you have successfully carried out all of the exercises described above before taking the self-test and before going to your instructor for the chapter evaluation exam. If you neglect these exercises, you will not be able to meet all the objectives for this chapter and may not receive a passing grade for this course.

Answers to Review Exercise A

1. (a) sternum   (b) clavicles   (c) scapulae
   (d) ribs   (e) thoracic vertebrae

2. Vertebra prominens (or spinous process of 7th cervical vertebra)

3. A. Jugular notch
   B. Manubrial notch or suprasternal notch

4. A. Larynx
   B. Trachea
   C. Right and left bronchi
   D. Lungs

5. A. Thyroid cartilage
   B. Larynx
   C. Sternum
   D. Scapula
   E. Clavicle

6. A. Nasopharynx
   B. Oropharynx
   C. Laryngopharynx

7. Epiglottis

8. Anteriorly

9. A. C3
   B. C6
   C. C5
   D. C6
   E. T4 or 5

10. Hyoid Bone

11. A. Right
    B. Because it is larger and more vertical in position

12. Carina

13. A. Right lung
    B. Upper, middle, lower lobes

14. Alveoli

15. A. Pleura
    B. Parietal pleura
    C. Pulmonary or visceral pleura
    D. Pleural cavity, pneumothorax

16. A. Base
    B. Hilus or hilum
    C. Apex

17. Mediastinum

18. A. Heart and great vessels
    B. Trachea
    C. Esophagus
    D. Thymus gland

19. A. Right
    B. Presence of the large liver in right upper abdomen

20. Costophrenic angle

21. B. Pharynx
    C. Larynx
    D. Trachea
    E. Bronchi, divided into primary or main stem bronchi and secondary bronchi

22. Pericardial sac

23. Left

If you missed more than 8 blanks, your score is less than 80% and you should review this section again in the textbook and/or audio-visuals before continuing.

Answers to Review Exercise B

1. A. Hypersthenic
   B. Asthenic
   C. Sthenic and hyposthenic

2. 10 (11 more common on healthy patients)

3. (a) low   (b) high

4. To be able to see faint outlines of vertebrae and posterior ribs through heart and mediastinal structures.

5. A. Possible small pneumothorax
   B. Fixation or lack of movement of diaphragm
   C. Presence of foreign body
   D. Distinguish between an opacity in the rib or in the lungs

6. A. To allow diaphragm to move down farther
   B. To show possible air and fluid levels
   C. To prevent engorgement and hyperemia (collection of fluid) in pulmonary vessels

7. To minimize magnification of heart and other structures in chest

8. Weight of abdominal organs will allow diaphragm to move down farther in erect position

9. To allow radiologist to determine amount of fluid present from air-fluid levels

10. A. Asymmetrical appearance of sternoclavicular joints, and/or unequal distances from the vertebral column to lateral borders of ribs
    B. Posterior ribs are not superimposed, and/or costophrenic angles are not superimposed

11. A. Left lateral
    B. Right lateral
    C. Left lateral

12. Prevent arms from superimposing upper lungs

13. A. Right or left marker placed on the patient's correct side in the upper corner of the cassette
    B. Left marker, upper cassette area, in front of patient
    C. Right marker, upper area of cassette, in front of patient

14. Lesser

15. A. 7" inferior to vertebra prominens (to T7)
    B. 8" inferior to vertebra prominens (to T7)
    C. 9" inferior to vertebra prominens (to T7 - T8)
    D. 3-4" inferior to jugular notch
    E. 4-5" inferior to jugular notch

16. Crosswise

17. Vertebra prominens

18. (a) caudal   (b) sternum

19. To prevent cutoff of lateral lung margins due to increased divergence of x-rays at a shorter SID

20. A. Left lateral decub (fluid on downside)
    B. Left lateral decub (air on upside)

21. LAO, 60°

22. PA and left lateral

23. A. AP supine
    B. Lateral decubitus
    C. AP Lordotic
       or 4th choice
       Obliques

24. (a) Anteriorly   (b) Because of divergent x-ray beam

If you missed more than 10 blanks, your score is less than 80% and you should review this section again in the textbook and/or audio-visuals before continuing.

Self-Test

My score = _____ %

Directions: Take this self-test only after completing all the review exercises and laboratory activities in this chapter. Complete directions including grading requirements are described in the front pages of this workbook and in the self-test of Chapter 1.

Test

There are 50 blanks. Each correct blank is worth 2 points.

Fill in the correct answers to the following: (Spelling is important so correct any misspellings as you grade this test.)

1. List the structures through which oxygen will pass as it travels from the nose and mouth to the distal aspects of the lungs where the O_2 and CO_2 are exchanged in the blood.

   A. pharynx

   B. larynx

   C. trachea

   D. bronchi

   E. alveoli

2. List three reasons why chest radiographs should be taken in an erect position whenever possible:

   A. more air space - lower diaphragms

   B. prevent engorgement of PULMONARY vessels

   C. check possible fluid or air levels

3. The name of the small bone from which the larynx is suspended: hyoid

4. Fill in the correct anatomical term for the following:

   A. Organ of voice larynx

   B. Adam's Apple thyroid cartilage

   C. Breastbone sternum

   D. Shoulder blade scapula

   E. Collar bone clavicle

5. A. Which lung is shorter right

   B. Why? to make room for the liver

6. List the four structures located in the mediastinum:

    A. _heart + GREAT VESSELS_

    B. _major vessels TRACHEA_

    C. _thymus GLAND_

    D. _esophagus_

7. A. Which bronchus will foreign objects such as food particles most likely enter? _right_

    B. Why? _larger diameter, less angle (more vertical)_

8. What structure normally prevents foreign objects such as food particles from entering the respiratory

    system? _epiglottis_

9. Is the esophagus located anteriorly or posteriorly to the trachea? _anterior POSTERIOR_

10. List the names of the lobes in each lung:

    A. Right lung (3) _upper, middle, lower_

    B. Left lung (2) _upper, lower_

11. Describe how rotation can be detected on the following radiographs:

    A. PA chest _unequal distance to ribs, unequal distance of_ _FROM VERTEBRAL COLUMN TO LATERAL BORDER OF RIBS_

    B. Lateral chest _posterior ribs, hemidiaphragms not superimp_ _COSTOPHRENIC ANGLES sternoclavicular_

12. The double-walled membrane or sac containing the lungs is the (a) _pleural cavity_,

    of which the lining of the thoracic cavity is the (b) _parietal pleura_,

    and the covering of the lungs is the (c) _visceral_ or _pulmonary pleura_

13. How many ribs should be demonstrated above the diaphragm on an optimal PA chest? _10_

14. Identify the bony landmarks which should be used for central ray location with the following:

    A. AP chest _thyroid cartilage_ _JUGULAR NOTCH_

    B. PA chest _vertebra prominens_

15. The superior portion of the lungs reaching above the clavicles is called the _apices_ _APEX_.

16. The thyroid cartilage is at the level of which vertebra? _C5_

17. How could you differentiate between the right and left hemidiaphragms on a lateral chest? _right_
    is higher

18. Are the anterior or posterior ribs in the highest position as demonstrated on a lateral chest radiograph?
    POSTERIOR

19. What is the correct term describing the extreme lateral points where the diaphragm meets the ribs?
Costophrenic angles

20. What is the term describing the area of the lungs where the primary bronchi enter the lungs? _hilum_

21. Name the prominence or ridge inside the trachea at the division into the right and left bronchi. _Carina_

22. At what vertebral level do the right and left bronchi bifurcate or divide? _____ T5 _or T4._

23. What is the structure with three divisions which serves as a common passageway for both food and air?
pharynx

24. What is a pneumothorax and what causes it to occur? _collapsed lung— air or_ OUTSIDE
~~fluid~~ in the pleural cavity

25. The double-walled sac enclosing the heart is the _pericardial sac_ .

26. Indicate the positions or projection(s) which should be taken for the following:

   A. Routine chest with no chest pain or symptoms _PA left lat._

   B. Oblique chest for demonstrating the heart _LAO 60°_

   C. Decubitus position for possible fluid in right lung _rt. lat decub._

   D. Decubitus position for possible air in right lung _left lat. decub_

27. Identify three conditions or pathologies suggesting the need for both inspiration and expiration PA chest radiographs.

   A. _pneumothorax_

   B. _foreign objects_

   C. _diaphragm does not move_

28. For a true lateral chest on a wide broad-shouldered patient, why does the patient need to be rotated slightly anteriorly? _to adjust for diffusion of beam_
   DIVERGENT X-RAY BEAM

Answers to Self-Test

1. A. Pharynx
   B. Larynx
   C. Trachea
   D. Bronchi (primary & secondary)
   E. Alveoli

2. A. To allow diaphragm to move down farther
   B. To demonstrate possible air and fluid levels
   C. To prevent engorgement and hyperemia (collection of fluid) in pulmonary vessels

3. Hyoid bone

4. A. Larynx
   B. Thyroid cartilage
   C. Sternum
   D. Scapula
   E. Clavicle

5. A. Right
   B. Presence of liver under right diaphragm

6. A. Heart and great vessels
   B. Trachea
   C. Esophagus
   D. Thymus gland

7. A. Right
   B. Because it is larger and more vertical in position

8. Epiglottis

9. Posteriorly

10. A. Upper, middle & lower lobes
    B. Upper and lower lobes

11. A. Symmetrical appearance of sternoclavicular joints, or unequal distances from the vertebral column to lateral borders of ribs
    B. Posterior ribs and costophrenic angles should be superimposed

12. (a) pleura
    (b) parietal pleura
    (c) pulmonary or visceral pleura

13. Minimum of 10

14. A. Jugular notch
    B. Vertebra prominens

15. Apex

16. C5

17. Right hemidiaphragm is higher

18. Posterior

19. Costophrenic angle

20. Hilus or hilum

21. Carina

22. T4 or 5

23. Pharynx

24. A condition of collapsed lung due to outside air filling the pleural cavity.

25. Pericardial sac

26. A. PA and left lateral
    B. LAO, 60° rotation
    C. Right lateral decubitus
    D. Left lateral decubitus

27. A. Possible small pneumothorax
    B. Fixation or lack of movement of diaphragm
    C. Presence of foreign body or 4th choice
       To distinguish between an opacity in the rib or in the lungs

28. Due to divergent x-ray beam

Chapter 3
Abdomen

Rationale

A very common radiographic examination is that of the abdomen, not only as an examination in itself, but also as an initial or scout radiograph for a number of routine and special procedures. The fact that many abdominal radiographs are taken during a given day in most radiology departments, makes this examination similar to the chest radiograph in the frequency of their performance. Care must be taken so that careless habits are not developed which will lead to less than optimal radiographs.

There are many organs representing several organ systems located within the abdominopelvic cavity so that a great deal of information can be obtained by the radiologist or the patient's physician, when they view the completed radiograph. Thus, it is necessary for the student and the technologist to have a thorough understanding of the abdominal organs as well as knowledge relating to their location in the various regions or quadrants of the abdomen.

The purpose of this chapter is to help you learn and understand both the anatomy and the standard positioning routines of the abdomen. Knowledge of the anatomy is essential if you are to understand the importance of routine views of the abdomen as well as a basis for future understanding of many more specialized procedures. In addition to learning how to position for the various views of the abdomen, you will learn how to view and critique abdominal radiographs to check for positioning accuracy and proper exposure factors.

Chapter Objectives

After you have successfully completed **all** the activities of this chapter, you will be able, with at least 80% accuracy, to: (applicable to a written and/or oral examination and demonstration)

___ 1. Identify both on drawings and radiographs the anatomy of the principal organs and structures of the **digestive system, liver** and **bilary system, pancreas, spleen**, and the **urinary system** and **adrenal glands**. The detail of important anatomy is defined in this chapter in the textbook and/or audio-visuals.

___ 2. Localize all organs as identified in objective 1 to one of the four quadrants of the abdomen.

___ 3. Identify and describe five bony positioning landmarks used for positioning abdominal radiographs and describe the relationship of these bony landmarks to other skeletal structures.

___ 4. List and describe the location of the three muscles of the abdomen important in abdominal radiography.

___ 5. Name and identify on drawings and radiographs those parts of the stomach, small intestine, large intestine, bile ducts and urinary system as identified in the textbook and/or the audio-visuals.

___ 6. Divide the abdomen into nine regions and name all regions.

___ 7. List and describe the four common variations in body habitus and describe the differences in shape and/or location of the stomach within these body types.

___ 8. List four types of pathology which would indicate need for a 3-way or acute abdomen series.

___ 9. Identify **which** lateral decubitus should be taken if there is a question of possible "free" air in the abdomen.

___ 10. Simulate taking supine, upright, and lateral decubitus abdominal radiographs on a phantom or a model posing as an ambulatory or stretcher patient.

Given several abdominal radiographs to view in supine, erect and lateral decubitus positions:

___ 11. Critique and evaluate each radiograph based on evaluation criteria provided in the textbook and/or audio-visuals.

___ 12. Identify all visible anatomical parts of the abdominopelvic cavity as identified in the textbook and/or audio-visuals.

___ 13. Discriminate between those radiographs which are acceptable and those which are unacceptable in centering and overall positioning, motion, definition and exposure factors for supine, erect and lateral decubitus positions.

___ 14. Discriminate between those radiographs which were taken in supine, erect or lateral decubitus positions.

Prerequisite Knowledge

The only prerequisite knowledge requirement for this chapter is an understanding of radiographic terminology and the principles of positioning as defined in Chapter 1. It is strongly suggested that a mandatory prerequisite for this chapter be the successful completion of Chapter 1 of this series. It is also suggested that completion of Chapter 2, "Radiographic Anatomy and Positioning of the Chest," would be helpful in understanding certain parts of this chapter but should not be a required prerequisite.

Recommended Supplementary References

The recommended supplementary references are listed to provide you with additional resources if you want more information on the material covered in this chapter. Even though all the information needed to meet the objectives of this chapter is provided in the Bontrager Textbook and/or the audio-visuals, it is suggested that at least one or two of the following references be read and studied for a more thorough understanding of this material. The following references, which are described in more detail in Chapter 1, are listed in a suggested order of importance and value to understanding this information.

1. *Merrill's ...*, Vol 2, pp 29-43

2. *Clark's...*, pp 309-324.

3. *Eisenberg ...*, pp 207-261

Learning Exercises

The following review exercises should be completed only after careful study of the associated pages in the textbook and/or the audio-visuals as indicated by each exercise.

After completing each of these individual exercises, check your answers with the answers provided at the end of the review exercises.

Part I. RADIOGRAPHIC ANATOMY

Review Exercise A   Abdominopelvic Anatomy   Textbook: pp 79-88
Audio-visuals: Unit 3, slides 1-29

1. Fill in the name of each anatomical part indicated by the letters in this drawing:

A. _iliac crest_

B. _ASIS (anterior superior iliac spine)_

C. _greater trochanter_

D. _ischial tuberosity_

E. _symphysis pubis_

F. _coccyx_

G. _sacrum_

H. _lumbar vertebra L5_

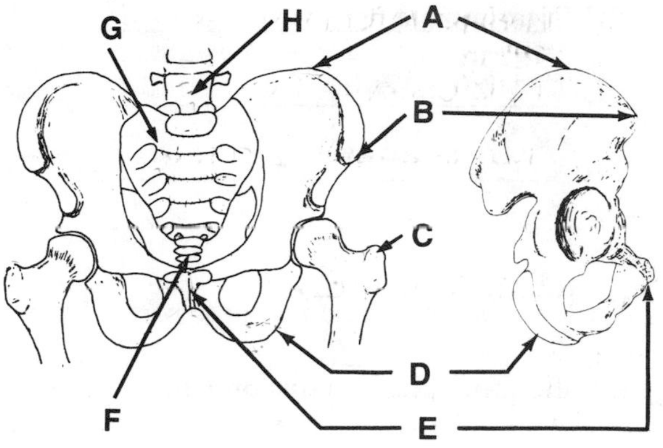

Fig. 3-1

2. The superior margin of the greater trochanter is about (a) _1-1½_ inches _superior_ (superior or inferior) to the level of the symphysis pubis, and the ischial tuberosity is about (b) _1½_ inches _inferior_ (superior or inferior) to the superior aspect of the symphysis pubis.

3. The crest of the ilium is at the level of _the disc space between 4L & 5L_ vertebra.

4. The name of the large muscles forming part of the posterior wall of the abdomen, the borders of which should be seen on abdominal radiographs? _psoas major - left & right_

5. The double-walled membrane lining the abdominal cavity is called the (a) _peritoneum_, of which the outer layer is the (b) _parietal peritoneum_, the inner layer is the (c) _visceral peritoneum_ and the double fold portion supporting certain organs is the (d) _mesentery_ or _omentum_.

6. Those organs located posteriorly to or behind this serous membrane lining the abdominopelvic cavity are referred to as being ___retroperitoneal___ .

7. Fill in the correct anatomical parts identified on this drawing of the stomach and small intestine:

A. cardiac orifice

B. fundus

C. body

D. rugae

E. pyloric antrum

F. pylorus   PYLORIC ORIFICE

G. duodenum

H. jejunum

I. ileum

J. ileocecal valve

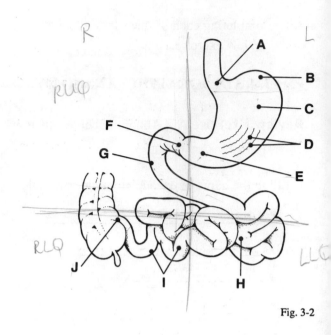

Fig. 3-2

8. Write in the correct name of the parts of the large intestine identified on this drawing:

A. cecum

B. ascending colon

C. R colic flexure (hepatic)

D. transverse colon

E. L colic flexure (splenic)

F. descending colon

G. sigmoid colon

H. rectum

I. anus

J. appendix

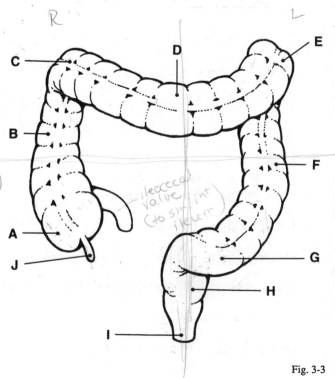

Fig. 3-3

9. The three accessory digestive organs are: A. _pancreas_

    B. _liver_   C. _gallbladder_

10. The liver is found in which quadrant of the abdomen? _right upper RUQ_

11. The pancreas is located anteriorly or posteriorly to the stomach? _posterior_

12. The tail of the pancreas is located in which quadrant of the abdomen? _upper left LUQ_

13. What is the organ of the circulatory system found in the left upper quadrant? _____

    spleen

14. List the parts of the organs identified on this drawing:

    A. _liver_

    B. _common hepatic duct_

    C. _common bile duct_

    D. _spleen_

    E. _pancreas_

    F. _duodenum_

    G. _sphincter of Oddi_

    H. _cystic duct_

    I. _gallbladder_

    J. _R hepatic duct_

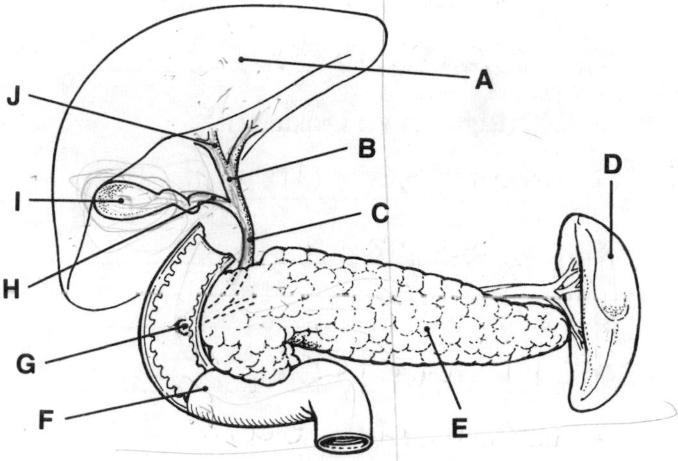

Fig. 3-4

15. Fill in correct parts of the urinary system as identified on this drawing.

    A. _left kidney_

    B. _left ureter_

    C. _urinary bladder_

    D. _urethra_

    E. _right adrenal gland_

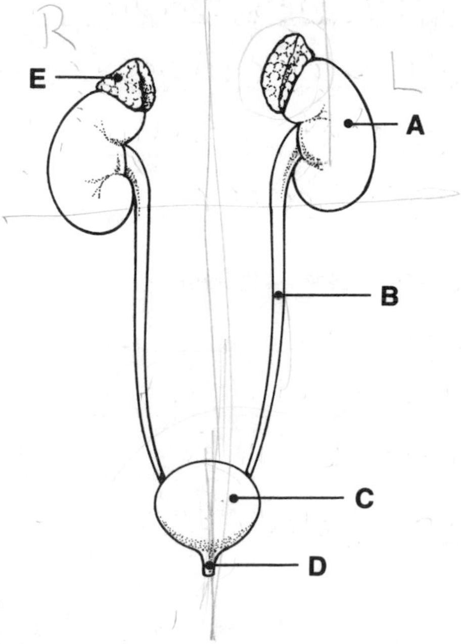

Fig. 3-5

16. The location of which organ of the upper right quadrant causes the right kidney to lie inferior to the left

kidney? _____liver_____

17. List those abdominopelvic organs or parts of organs and structures located in each of the four quadrants: (The drawings of the abdomen in Figures 3-6 and 3-7 on the following page may be helpful in remembering which parts are in each of these four quadrants.)

A. R.U.Q. (Right Upper Quadrant)
1. liver
2. gallbladder
3. rt. kidney
4. rt. adrenal gland
5. head of pancreas
6. C-loop of duodenum
7. part of jejunum
8. R. colic flexure of colon
9. R. transverse colon

B. R.L.Q. (Right Lower Quadrant)
1. lower ascending colon
2. cecum
3. appendix
4. rt. ureter
5. terminal ileum
6. half of rectum
7. half of urinary bladder
8. rt. psoas major muscle
9. ileocecal valve

C. L.L.Q. (Left Lower Quadrant)
1. lower descending colon
2. sigmoid colon
3. part of ileum
4. left ureter
5. half of rectum
6. half of urinary bladder
7. left psoas major muscle

D. L.U.Q. (Left Upper Quadrant)
1. spleen
2. stomach
3. left kidney
4. left adrenal gland
5. L colic (splenic) flexure
6. tail of pancreas
7. part of jejunum
8. left transverse colon

18. Write in the names of the **nine** regions of the abdomen.

(1) _R hypochondriac_

(2) _epigastric_

(3) _L hypochondriac_

(4) _R lateral_

(5) _umbilical_

(6) _L lateral_

(7) _R inguinal_

(8) _pubic_

(9) _L inguinal_

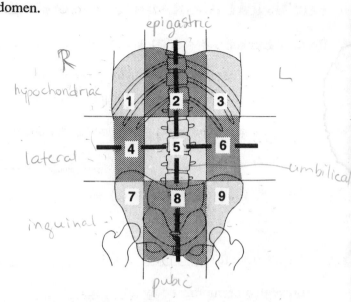

Fig. 3-6

19. Identify the four common variations in body habitus and the approximate percent of the population comprising each type.

A. _hypersthenic_ , _5_ %   C. _hyposthenic_ , _35_ %

B. _sthenic_ , _50_ %   D. _asthenic_ , _10_ %

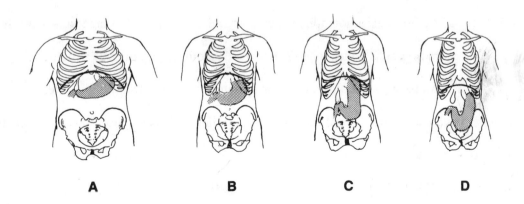

A   B   C   D

20. Which body habitus may require two cassettes placed crosswise to insure that the lateral margins of the abdomen are not cut off? _hypersthenic_

21. For which two body types comprising nearly 50% of the population is the stomach location lower and more <u>vertical</u> in position? (a) _hyposthenic_ (b) _asthenic_

Part II. RADIOGRAPHIC POSITIONING

Review Exercise B   Shielding Considerations, Exposure Factors and Positioning

Textbook: pp 89-97
Audio-visuals: Unit 3, slides 30-50

1. Motion is a serious detriment to good abdominal radiographs. Voluntary motion for the abdomen primarily

   results from (a)_____ breathing _____.

   Two ways to prevent it are to (b)_____ proper instructions _____ and

   (c)_____ short exposure time _____. Involuntary motion

   results from (d)_____ peristalsis _____ and can be

   prevented or minimized by (e)_____ short ~~quick~~ exposure _____.

2. True or False: Four sided collimation borders of at least a half inch inside film margins should **always** be

   visible on abdominal radiographs for all adult patients? _____ false _____

3. True or False: A. Gonadal shielding should **always** be used when taking abdomen radiographs of males

              of childbearing age or younger. _____ true _____

            B. Gonadal shielding should **always** be used when taking abdomen radiographs of females

              of childbearing age or younger. _____ false _____

4. True or False: A. Abdominal radiographs generally require a lower kVp range to produce high contrast

              radiographs which best visualize all abdominal organs and structures. _____ ~~true~~ false-mod

            B. A moving or stationary grid is required for a routine adult abdomen. _____ true _____

5. A good way to evaluate an abdominal radiograph for sufficient density, based on soft tissue differentiation

   on an average size adult patient, is to be able to visualize the borders of certain organs and structures.

   Name these: (a)_____ psoas muscles _____ (b)_____ lower liver _____

   (c)_____ kidney outlines _____, and (d)_____ lumbar vertebrae transverse proces[s]

6. A. If you were asked to take a KUB film, what would you radiograph and in what position would you

              place the patient? _____ AP supine abdomen _____

   B. For what do the initials KUB stand? _____ kidneys - ureters - bladder _____

7. Give two reasons why a PA chest is frequently included as part of an acute abdomen series.

    A. _to see free air_

    B. _some chest diseases have abdominal pain_

8. Which two projections of the abdomen best demonstrate air-fluid levels and free intra-abdominal air?

    A. _AP erect_   and/or _left lat decubitus_

    B. Why these two projections? _air will go to the top - horizontal beam_

9. Which lateral decubitus best demonstrates free intra-abdominal air? (right or left lateral decubitus)

    A. _left_

    B. Why? _air goes to the top (rt. side)_

10. What is the advantage of taking an abdomen PA rather than AP on a young female patient when the kidneys are not of primary interest? _less exposure to reprod. organs_

11. A national survey (as quoted in textbook) indicates in the United States there are four projections commonly taken for an acute abdomen series. Rank in order these four projections from the highest frequency to the lowest:

    A. _AP supine_

    B. _AP ~~supine~~ erect_

    C. _PA chest_

    D. _lat decub._

12. If the patient is too weak to sit or stand for an erect chest or abdomen on an acute abdomen series, what two projections should be taken as a minimum?

    A. _left lat. decubitus_

    B. _AP supine_

13. To what level should one center an average adult erect or decubitus abdominal film in order to include the diaphragm? _2" above iliac crest_

14. List the four most common indications associated with acute abdomen series requests:

A. _perforated hollow viscus_

B. _bowel obstruction_

C. _Infection_

D. _intra-abdominal mass_

15. In addition to the four projections commonly taken as part of an acute abdomen series, which projection or positions should be taken to demonstrate a possible aneurysm or calcification of the aorta or other major vessel?

dorsal decubitus

16. What respiratory phase should be routinely employed for abdominal radiography (inspiration or expiration)? _expiration_

exp - supine

insp - upright

Review Exercise C   Laboratory Activity   Textbook: pp 91-97

This part of the learning activity exercise series needs to be carried out in a radiographic laboratory or a general diagnostic room in a radiology department with facilities for a 3-way abdominal series.

Positioning Exercise

For this section you need another person to act as your "patient" and you should go through ALL the steps (except making exposure) as outlined in the textbook and/or audio visuals. Practice the following until you can do each of them accurately and without hesitation. Place a check by each when you have achieved this.

Include the following details as you simulate each of the following projections/positions:

- correct placement of film holder
- correct placement of marker
- correct patient positioning
- correct placement of lead shields
- correct CR location and collimation
- approximate correct exposure technique
- correct breathing instructions as you simulate the exposure

___ 1. Simulate taking an AP supine abdominal radiograph. Include all steps from the time the "patient walks in the door until the exposure is "made."

___ 2. Simulate positioning for an erect and a lateral decubitus abdomen. Include correct positioning, film placement with markers and tube alignment with accurate collimation.

___ 3. Simulate positioning for a PA prone abdomen.

___ 4. Simulate positioning for a dorsal decubitus abdomen.

Optional

___ 5. If a full-body phantom is available, take a KUB abdomen and produce a satisfactory radiograph with correct positioning and correct technical factors including density, contrast, and film marker placement.

Review Exercise D Film Critique and Evaluation   Textbook: pp 91-97

Your instructor will provide various abdominal radiographs for these exercises. These should include AP supine, erect, lateral decubitus and dorsal decubitus, some of which should be optimum quality radiographs based on evaluation criteria provided for each projection in the textbook and/or audio-visuals. Several should be unacceptable requiring a repeat exam and others should be less than optimum quality as to positioning, exposure factors, collimation errors and/or patient ID or marker placement.

Place a check by each of the following when it is completed.

__ 1. Determine in which body position each of these radiographs were taken, supine, erect, or lateral decubitus.

__ 2. Critique each radiograph based on evaluation criteria provided for each projection in the textbook and/or audio-visuals. The following criteria guidelines can be used and checked as each radiograph is evaluated.

         Radiographs   Criteria Guidelines

     1   2   3   4   5   6

     __   __   __   __   __   __   a. Transverse (side-to-side) centering?

     __   __   __   __   __   __   b. Lengthwise (top-to-bottom) centering?

     __   __   __   __   __   __   c. Correct collimation?

     __   __   __   __   __   __   d. Rotation?

     __   __   __   __   __   __   e. Motion?

     __   __   __   __   __   __   f. Exposure: density, and/or contrast?

     __   __   __   __   __   __   g. Patient ID information and markers?

__ 3. Based on acceptable variances to criteria factors, determine which of these radiographs are acceptable and which are unacceptable and should have been repeated.

Answers to Review Exercise A

1. A. Iliac crest or crest of ilium
   B. Anterior superior iliac spine, or ASIS
   C. Greater trochanter of femur
   D. Ischial tuberosity
   E. Symphysis pubis
   F. Coccyx
   G. Sacrum
   H. L5 (fifth lumbar vertebra)

2. (a) 1.5 inches superior to (b) 1.5 inches inferior to

3. Disc space between L4 and L5

4. Right and left major psoas muscles

5. (a) Peritoneum (b) Parietal peritoneum
   (c) Visceral peritoneum (d) Mesentery
   or omentum

6. Retroperitoneal structures

7. A. Cardiac orifice
   B. Fundus
   C. Body
   D. Rugae
   E. Pyloric antrum
   F. Pyloric orifice
   G. Duodenum
   H. Jejunum
   I. Ileum
   J. Ileocecal valve

8. A. Cecum
   B. Ascending colon
   C. R. colic (hepatic) flexure
   D. Transverse colon
   E. L. colic (splenic) flexure
   F. Descending colon
   G. Sigmoid colon
   H. Rectum
   I. Anus
   J. Appendix

9. A. Liver B. Gallbladder C. Pancreas

10. Right upper quadrant (RUQ)

11. Posterior

12. Left upper quadrant (LUQ)

13. Spleen

14. A. Liver
    B. Common hepatic duct
    C. Common bile duct
    D. Spleen
    E. Pancreas
    F. Duodenum
    G. Sphincter of Oddi
    H. Cystic duct
    I. Gallbladder
    J. Right hepatic duct

15. A. Left kidney
    B. Left ureter
    C. Urinary bladder
    D. Urethra
    E. Right adrenal gland

16. Liver

17. A. 1. Liver
       2. Gallbladder
       3. Right kidney
       4. Right adrenal gland
       5. Head of pancreas
       6. C-loop of duodenum
       7. Part of jejunum
       8. R. colic flexure of colon
       9. Right transverse colon

    B. 1. Lower ascending colon
       2. Cecum
       3. Appendix
       4. Right ureter
       5. Terminal ileum
       6. Half of rectum
       7. Half of urinary bladder
       8. Right psoas major muscle
       9. Ileocecal valve

    C. 1. Lower descending colon
       2. Sigmoid colon
       3. Part of ileum
       4. Left ureter
       5. Half of rectum
       6. Half of urinary bladder
       7. Left psoas major muscle

    D. (next page)

Answers to Review Exercise A continued

D. 1. Spleen
   2. Stomach
   3. Left kidney
   4. Left adrenal
   5. L colic (splenic) flexure of colon
   6. Tail of pancreas
   7. Part of jejunum
   8. Left transverse colon

18. (1) Right hypochondriac region
    (2) Epigastric region
    (3) Left hypochondriac region
    (4) Right lateral (lumbar) region
    (5) Umbilical region
    (6) Left lateral (lumbar) region
    (7) Right inguinal (iliac) region
    (8) Pubic (hypogastric) region
    (9) Left inguinal (iliac) region

19. A. Hypersthenic,   5%
    B. Sthenic,   50%
    C. Hyposthenic,   35%
    D. Asthenic,   10%

20. Hypersthenic

21. (a) Hyposthenic
    (b) Asthenic

If you missed more than 22 blanks, you should
review this section again in the textbook and/or
audio-visuals before continuing.

Answers to Review Exercise B

1. (a) Breathing movements during exposure, (b) Give careful breathing instructions and (c) Use short exposure times. (d) Peristaltic action of bowel, (e) Use of the shortest exposure time possible.

2. False (Collimation should be only to actual film border on most adult patients so as not to cut off essential anatomy, especially on top and bottom borders.)

3. A. True
   B. False (only if such ovarian shields do not cover essential abdominopelvic anatomy)

4. A. False (medium kVp should be used for moderate contrast)
   B. True

5. (a) psoas muscles (b) lower liver margin (c) kidney outlines (d) lumbar vertebrae transverse processes

6. A. AP abdomen, patient supine
   B. Kidneys, Ureters, Bladder

7. A. Best visualizes possible free air under diaphragm
   B. Certain chest diseases are frequently associated with severe abdominal pain

8. A. Lateral decubitus erect
   B. A horizontal beam is used.

9. A. Left (patient on left side)
   B. Free air rises and is best demonstrated in the area of the liver.

10. PA results in significantly less gonadal dose on females.

11. A. AP supine   C. PA chest
    B. AP erect   D. Lateral decubitus

12. A. AP supine abdomen   B. Left lateral decubitus

13. 2" superior to iliac crest

14. A. Perforated hollow viscus (free intra-abdominal air)
    B. Bowel obstruction
    C. Infection
    D. Intra-abdominal mass

15. Dorsal decubitus position

16. Expiration

If you missed more than 7 blanks, you should review this section again in the textbook and/or audio-visuals before continuing.

Self-Test

My score = _____ %

Directions: Take this self-test only after completing all the review exercises and laboratory activities in this chapter. Complete directions including grading requirements are described in the front pages of this workbook and in the self-test of Chapter 1.

Test

There are 65 blanks, so each correct blank is worth 1.5 points. (Spelling is important so correct any mis-spellings as you grade your test.)

1. The crest of the ilium is at the level of what vertebral anatomy? _L5_ _L4-L5_

2. The prominent anterior spine of the crest is termed the _ASIS_ _anterior superior iliac spine_ .

3. The anterior junction of the two pubic bones is the _symphysis pubis_ .

4. Describe the relationship in position of the superior margin of the greater trochanter to the symphysis pubis. _1½ inches superior to symphysis pubis_   _ISCHIAL TUBEROSITY 1½" below S.P._

5. The term describing those organs located posterior to the serous membrane lining the abdominopelvic cavity: _retroperitoneal_

6. This muscle separates the thoracic cavity from the abdominopelvic cavity. _diaphragm_

7. Identify the parts of this drawing:

   A. _esophagus_

   B. _cardiac orifice_

   C. _LESSER CURVATURE_

   D. _duodenum_

   E. _pyloric orifice_

   F. _pyloric antrum_

   G. _rugae_

   H. _body GREATER CURVATURE_

   I. _BODY_

   J. _fundus_

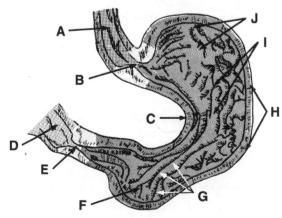

Fig. 3-8

8. This pair of muscles should be seen on the AP abdominal radiograph to each side of the lumbar vertebral column. _L + R psoas major_

9. Identify the labeled parts of the small bowel.

A. _duodenum_

B. _ileocecal valve_

C. _ileum_

D. _jejunum_

E. _pyloric orifice_

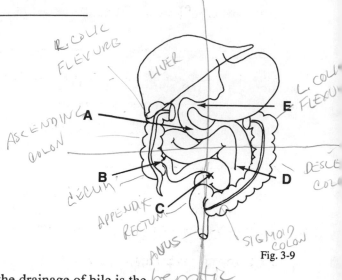

Fig. 3-9

10. The **main** duct leading directly from the liver for the drainage of bile is the _hepatic_ duct.

11. The duct leading directly from the gall bladder is the _bile_ _cystic_ duct.

12. The above two ducts join to form the _COMMON BILE DUCT_ which connects to the duodenum.

13. The opening into the duodenum of the above duct is called _SPHINCTER OF ODDI_.

14. Identify the labeled parts of the large intestine.

A. _transverse colon_

B. _R. colic flexure_

C. _ascending colon_

D. _ileocecal valve_

E. _cecum_

F. _appendix_

G. _anus_

H. _rectum_

I. _sigmoid colon_

J. _descending colon_

K. _L colic flexure_

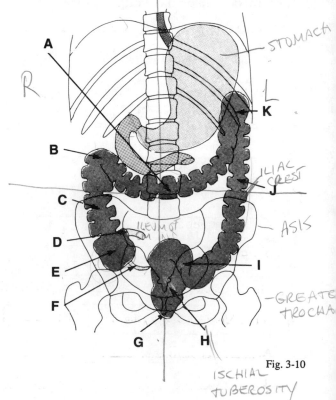

Fig. 3-10

15. If an abdominal examination is ordered on a patient with a diagnosis of possible bowel obstruction and

the patient is **very** weak and cannot sit up, what view(s) would you take?

L. lat decub   AP supine

16. What is the name of the tube-like structure leading from the urinary bladder to the exterior of the body?

urethra

17. What is the name of the tube-like structure leading from the kidney to the urinary bladder?

ureters

18. A pair of important endocrine glands located atop the kidneys are the _adrenal_ .

19. Use initials to indicate the correct abdominal quadrant in which the following structures or organs are

usually found. (Indicate the quadrant in which the **major portion** of the organs or structures are normally

located on an average sthenic type patient.)

A. C-loop of duodenum   _LUQ RUP_   H. Left adrenal gland   _LUQ_

B. Cecum   _RUQ RLQ_   I. Gall bladder   _RUQ_

C. Sigmoid colon   _LLQ_   J. Right ureter   _RLQ_

D. Appendix   _RLQ_   K. Terminal ilium   _RUQ RLQ_

E. Liver   _RUQ_   L. Left colix flexure   _LUQ_

F. Stomach (body and fundus)   _LUQ_   M. Spleen   _LUQ_

G. Right kidney   _RUQ_   N. Pancreas (tail)   _LUQ_
       head = RUQ

20. Two horizontal planes and two vertical planes divide the abdomen into _nine_ regions.

21. An abdominal radiograph is usually taken with the patient holding his or her breath on _expiration_.

22. What bony landmarks should be used to position for an AP supine abdomen?

A. For center of film _iliac crest_

B. For lower margin of film _symphysis pubis_

23. The stomach is more transverse and is located high in the abdomen (usually above the iliac crest) on

about 55% of the population. Which two body habitus types are these?

A. _HYPERSTHENIC_

B. _STHENIC_

24. What is the centering point (CROSSWAYS) for an abdominal radiograph of an average sthenic type patient if it were necessary to include both hemidiaphragms on the finished radiograph?

_____sternum_____ 2" ABOVE ILIAC CREST_____

25. Which lateral decubitus abdomen would be taken if there were a question of free air from a perforated peptic ulcer? _____left_____

26. An air-fluid level would not be seen radiographically on which of the following projections: (1) Erect or upright abdomen; (2) left or right lateral decubitus abdomen; or (3) prone or supine abdomen.

_____3_____

27. List the four types of pathology which would indicate a need for a (3-way) or acute abdominal series:

A. _perforated bowel_   PA chest

B. _bowel obstruction_   AP abdomen supine

C. _abdominal mass_   AP abdomen upright (erect

D. _free air_   INFECTION

28. List those structures which should be faintly visible (in reference to soft tissue differentiation) on a correctly exposed radiograph of the abdomen:

A. _psoas muscles_

B. _lower liver_

C. _kidneys_

D. _vertebra - transverse processes_

Answers to Self-Test

1. Disc space between L4 and L5

2. Anterior superior iliac spine (ASIS)

3. Symphysis pubis

4. 1 or 1.5 inches above symphysis pubis

5. Retroperitoneal

6. Diaphragm

7. Right and left psoas muscles

8. A. Esophagus

   B. Esophagastric junction (cardiac orifice)

   C. Lesser curvature

   D. Small intestine (duodenum)

   E. Pyloric orifice (pylorus)

   F. Pyloric Antrum

   G. Rugae

   H. Greater curvature

   I. Body

   J. Fundus

9. A. Duodenum

   B. Ileocecal valve

   C. Ileum

   D. Jejunum

   E. Pyloric orifice

10. Common hepatic

11. Cystic

12. Common bile

13. The Sphincter of Oddi

14. A. Transverse colon

   B. R colic (hepatic) flexure

   C. Ascending colon

   D. Ileocecal valve

   E. Cecum

   F. Appendix

14. G. Anus

   H. Rectum

   I. Sigmoid colon

   J. Descending colon

   K. L colic (splenic) flexure

15. Supine and lateral decubitus

16. Urethra

17. Ureter

18. Adrenals

19. A. RUQ

   B. RLQ

   C. LLQ

   D. RLQ

   E. RUQ

   F. LUQ

   G. RUQ

20. Nine

21. Expiration

22. A. Iliac Crest

   B. Symphysis pubis or greater trochanter

23. A. Hypersthenic

   B. Sthenic

24. About 2 inches superior to iliac crest

25. Left lateral

26. (3) Prone or supine abdomen

27. A. Perforated viscus

   B. Intestinal obstruction

   C. Infection

   D. Intra-abdominal mass

28. A. Psoas muscles

   B. Kidney outlines

   C. Lower border of liver

   D. Transverse processes of lumbar vertebrae

Chapter 4
Upper Limb

Thumb, Fingers, Hand, Wrist, Forearm, Elbow and Humerus

Rationale

If you as a student are to achieve accuracy and consistency in radiographing the upper limb, you must develop a good understanding of the relationship between various anatomical parts. You must know the correct central ray locations as well as the correct positioning views, angles, and rotations. You should also understand why certain positions and certain central ray locations are important so you can remember these and make modifications if the condition of the patient is such that you can't do the usual routines.

You must be able to critique the radiographs you have taken to know what errors you have made and must know how these errors can be corrected. You must also know which anatomical parts need to be visualized and must be able to critique films to see if these parts are all visualized well. You will learn how to evaluate radiographs for accuracy of positioning and exposure factors utilizing specific evaluation criteria.

If you have a good knowledge of the anatomy and the relationships between anatomical parts, you will be able to correctly position certain "non-routine" views if such are requested by the referring physician. You should know and understand the anatomy and relationships well enough to be able to suggest which special projections could be taken to best visualize the area of interest.

Successful completion of all the exercises in this chapter should provide you with enough knowledge and skill to perform actual radiographic examinations of the upper limb on patients under the supervision of a technologist.

Chapter Objectives

After you have successfully completed **all** the activities of this chapter, you will be able, with at least 80% accuracy, to: (applicable to a written and/or oral examination and demonstration)

___ 1. Identify on drawings, radiographs, and on a dry skeleton all anatomy of the upper limb as described in this chapter in the textbook and/or audio-visuals.

___ 2. List more than one name for the carpals where so indicated.

___ 3. Identify by name and by classification and movement type all joints of the upper limb as described in the textbook and/or audio-visuals.

___ 4. For all basic and optional projections, list the technical factors and the central ray locations for the **thumb, fingers, hand, wrist, forearm, elbow** and **humerus**.

___ 5. Position on a model or phantom all basic and optional projections for each upper limb examination.

___   6.   List the basic projections usually taken for a limb in a cast and the approximate exposure conversion guidelines.

___   7.   Describe the basic projections which should be taken for a partially flexed elbow which cannot be extended.

___   8.   Describe the projections or positions which would best demonstrate each of the following specific anatomical parts: **head** and **neck** of radius, **coronoid process** of ulna, **olecranon process** of ulna and **relationship of head of humerus to glenoid fossa.**

___   9.   Critique radiographs based on evaluation criteria provided in the textbook and/or audio-visuals.

___   10.   Discriminate between radiographs which are acceptable and those which are unacceptable due to exposure factors, collimation or positioning errors.

Prerequisite

The only prerequisite knowledge requirement for this chapter is an understanding of radiographic terminology and the principles of exposure, radiation protection, and positioning as described in Chapter 1. It is strongly suggested that a mandatory prerequisite for this chapter be the successful completion of Chapter 1.

Recommended Supplementary References

The following supplementary references, which are described in more detail in Chapter 1, are listed in a suggested order of importance and value to understanding this material.

1.   *Merrill's ...*, Vol 1, pp 51-109

2.   *Clark's ...*, pp 34-67

3.   *Eisenberg ...*, pp 37-76

Learning Exercises

The following review exercises should be completed only after careful study of the associated pages in the textbook and/or audio-visuals as indicated by each exercise.

After completing each of these individual exercises, check your answers with the answer sheets which follow before continuing to the next exercise.

Part I. RADIOGRAPHIC ANATOMY

Review Exercise A   Anatomy of Hand and Wrist   Textbook: pp 99-103
                                             Audio-visuals, Unit 4, slides 1-17

1. Fill in the number of bones in the following:

   A. Phalanges (fingers and thumb) __14__

   B. Metacarpals (palm) __5__

   C. Carpals (wrist) __8__

   D. Total __27__

2. List the two bones making up the 1st digit (thumb):

   A. ~~1st metacarpal~~ proximal phalanx   B. distal phalanx

3. The joint between the above two bones is called the ~~metacarpophalangeal~~ interphalangeal joint.

4. Fill in the following bones and joints from this drawing of the right hand:

   A. 1st metacarpal

   B. metacarpophalangeal joint

   C. proximal phalanx of 1st digit

   D. interphalangeal joint

   E. middle phalanx of 2nd digit

   F. distal phalanx of 3rd digit

   G. DISTAL interphalangeal joint

   H. PROXIMAL interphalangeal joint

   I. proximal ~~middle~~ phalanx of 5th digit

   J. 5th metacarpophalangeal joint

   K. 5th metacarpal

   L. carpometacarpal joint

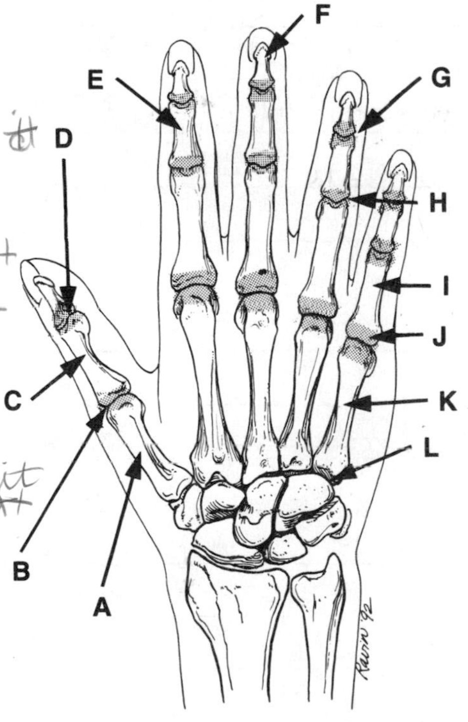

Fig. 4-1

5. Write in the names of the carpals, giving the preferred name first and the second or third name where indicated (hint—use the mnemonic given in the textbook):

Proximal row, starting from lateral (thumb) side

A. _scaphoid_ (_navicular_)
B. _lunate_ (_semilunar_)
C. _triquetrum_ (_triangular_ or _cuneiform_)
D. _pisiform_

Distal row, starting from lateral side

E. _trapezium_ (_greater multangular_)
F. _trapezoid_ (_lesser multangular_)
G. _capitate_ (_os magnum_)
H. _hamate_ (_unciform_)

6. Which is the largest of the carpal bones? _capitate_

7. Which of the carpals has a "hook-like" process extending anteriorly which can be readily palpated?
(a) _hamate_ What is the name of the process? (b) _hamulus_

8. Which carpal is most commonly fractured? _scaphoid_

9. Identify the parts of these frontal and carpal canal views of the right wrist (use preferred names of carpals):

A. _lunate_
B. _triquetrum_
C. _pisiform_
D. _hamate_
E. _capitate_
F. _trapezoid_
G. _trapezium_
H. _scaphoid_

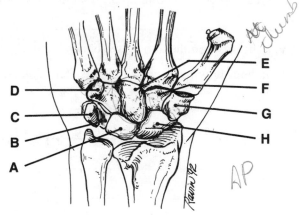

Fig. 4-2

I. _thumb 1st metacarpal_
J. _trapezium_
K. _trapezoid_
L. _capitate_
M. _hamate_
N. _pisiform_
O. _triquetrum_

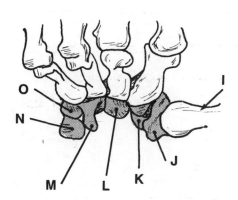

Fig. 4-3

Review Exercise B   Anatomy of the Forearm, Elbow and Distal humerus

Textbook: pp 104-108
Audio-visuals: Unit 5, slides 1-16

1. In the anatomical position, which of the bones of the forearm is located on the lateral side (thumb side)?
    (a)_ radius _____, and which is on the medial side? (b) _ ulna _____.

2. Fill in the following parts from this drawing of the left
    proximal ulna (lateral view):

    A. _ radial notch _(lateral)

    B. _corohoid tubercle_(medial)

    C._corohoid process_____

    D. _trochlear notch_____   SEMELWAR NOTCH

    E. _olecranon process_

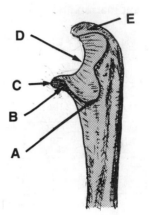

Fig. 4-4

3. Identify the labeled parts of this right forearm (anterior view):

    A._styloid process_____

    B. _radius_____(lateral bone of forearm)

    C. _shaft (body)_____

    D. _radial tuberosity_

    E. _neck_____

    F. _head_____

    G. _shaft (body)_

    H. _ulna_____(medial bone of forearm)

    I. _ulnar notch_

    J. _head_____

    K. _styloid process_

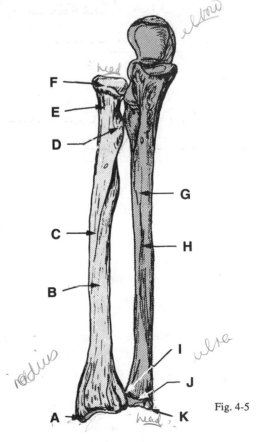

Fig. 4-5

4. The ulnar notch at the distal forearm is part of which bone of the forearm? _radius_

5. Which of the bones of the forearm articulates most directly with the carpal bones at the wrist joint?

    radius

6. Which of the bones of the forearm articulates most directly with the humerus at the elbow joint?

    ulna

7. The movements of supination and pronation of the forearm and hand are the result of the action of which

    two joints? (a) _proximal radio-ulnar_ and (b) _distal radio-ulnar_

8. Identify the labeled parts of this drawing of an AP right elbow:

    A. _radius_

    B. _head of radius_

    C. _capitulum_

    D. _lateral epicondyle_

    E. _radial fossa_

    F. _coronoid fossa_

    G. _medial condyle_

    H. _humeral condyle_

    I. _trochlea_

    J. _trochlea sulcus_

    K. _ulna_

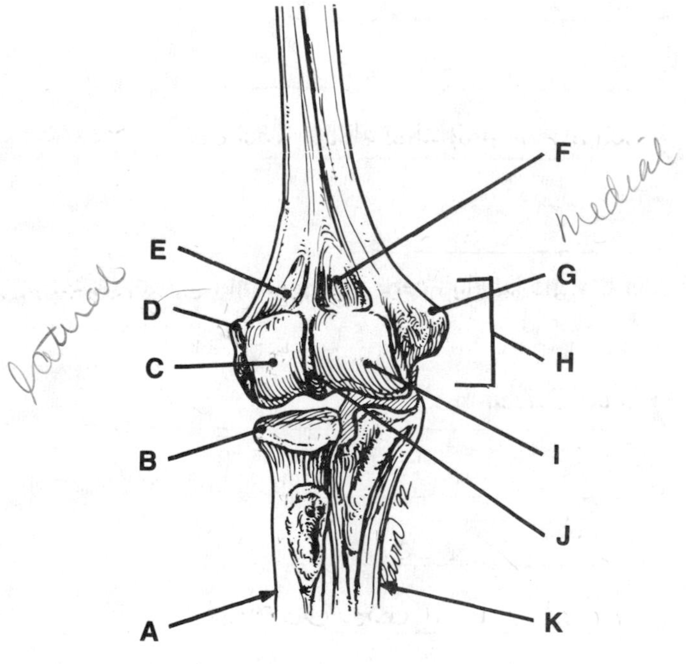

Fig. 4-6

9. The preferred term for the area of the distal humerus directly superior to the radial head is

    (a) _capitulum_ , the older or secondary term is (b) _capitellum_ .

10. Which of the two epicondyles of the distal humerus is the largest, the medial or lateral? _medial_

11. The two anterior depressions of the distal humerus are the (a) _radial fossa_ and

    (b) _coronoid fossa_ , and the deep posterior depression is the (c) _olecranon fossa_

12. A criteria for evaluating a good lateral elbow
    (when flexed 90°) is the appearance of three concentric
    or uniform arcs. Identify these from this drawing:

    A. trochlear sulcus

    B. outer ridges of trochlea + capitulum

    C. trochlear notch of ulna

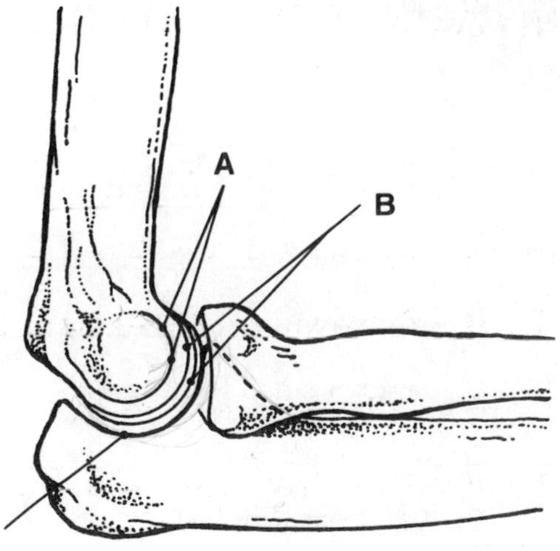

Fig. 4-7

13. Which flexion projection of the wrist best demonstrates the scaphoid (the radial or ulnar flexion)?

    (a) ulnar flexion   radial deviation   Which best demonstrates the lunate, triquetrum and pisiform?

    (b) radial flexion

14. What is a second term for the ulnar flexion wrist movement? radial deviation

15. Why should the forearm not be taken as a PA? rotation of the radius + ulna   crossover

16. Joint classifications:

    A. What is the **structural classification** of all joints of the upper limb studied in this chapter?

       synovial

    B. What is the **mobility classification** for all of these joints? diarthroid

    C. Identify the **movement types** for each of the following:

       1. Proximal and distal radioulnar joints? condyloid pivot

       2. Elbow (humeroulnar) joint? hinge

       3. All interphalangeal joints? hinge

       4. First metacarpophalangeal joint? saddle

       5. Second-fifth MP joints? condyloid

       6. First carpometacarpal joint? saddle

       7. Second-fifth CM joint? gliding

       8. All intercarpal joints? gliding

       9. Radiocarpal (wrist) joint? condyloid

Part II RADIOGRAPHIC POSITIONING

Review Exercise C   Positioning of the Fingers, Thumb, Hand and Wrist

Textbook: pp 109-129
Audio-visuals: Unit 4, slides 18-45

1. Fill in the following technical factors most commonly used for upper limb radiography:

   A. kVp range? _____ 50-70 _____ low-med

   B. Exposure time? _____ short _____

   C. Large or small focal spot? _____ small _____

   D. Most common SID? _____ 40" _____

   E. When are grids used? _____ body part more than 10cm. _____

   F. Type of film holder most commonly used? _____ intensifying screen/detail screen _____

   G. With small to medium dry plaster cast, increase _____ 5-7 _____ kVp.

   H. With large or wet plaster cast, increase (a) _____ 8-10 _____ kVp or (b) _____ double _____ mAs.

   I. With fiberglass cast, increase _____ 3-4 _____ kVp.

   J. Adequate mAs should be used for sufficient density to visualize (a) _____ soft tissue margins _____ and (b) _____ fine trabecular markings _____

2. A. The collimation rule which should be followed states: _____ borders should be evident on all 4 sides _____

   B. How can a radiograph be evaluated for correct CR location if four-sided collimation is   draw X corner to

   evident? _____ 90° or perpendicular to plane of cassette, directed to correct centering point _____

3. Gonad shielding for upper limbs should be used on all persons who are _____ of reproductive age _____

4. List the correct CR location for the following:

   A. Thumb _____ metacarpophalangeal joint _____ 1st MP joint

   B. Finger _____ proximal interphalangeal joint _____ PIP joint

   C. PA and Oblique hand _____ 3rd MP joint _____

   D. "Fan" lateral hand _____ 1st MP joint 2nd _____

   E. PA and Oblique wrist _____ midcarpal area _____

   F. PA wrist in ulnar flexion _____ scaphoid - navicular _____

4. *(continued)*

   G. Carpal canal view _1" distal to base of 3rd metacarpal_

   H. Carpal bridge view _midpoint of distal forearm 1½" prox. to wrist joint_

5. What is one important difference in basic projections between the thumb and fingers? _____

   fingers PA   thumb AP

6. What are two ways motion can be avoided?

   A. _short exposure time_

   B. _immobilization_

7. Starting in the prone (palm down) position, indicate which rotation of hand and wrist is needed for the following (**medial, lateral,** or **none**):

   A. Oblique thumb   _none_

   B. Lateral thumb   _medial_

   C. Oblique of 2nd digit   _medial_

   D. Oblique of 3rd digit   _lateral_

   E. Oblique of 4th digit   _lateral_

   F. Oblique of 5th digit   _lateral_

8. Why is it especially important to use a support block for an oblique hand? _prevents_
   to prevent motion
   foreshortening of phalanges + obscuring IP joints

9. How much should kVp be increased from a PA to a lateral hand? ___ _4-5_ ___

10. What degree of rotation is needed for an oblique hand? ___ _45°_ ___

11. What is the most common optional projection taken if the scaphoid is the primary area of interest?

   ulnar flexion PA   _navicular_

12. How much, in which direction, and why is the CR angled for the above optional projection (question 11)?

   A. Degrees of angle? _15-20°_

   B. Direction of angle? _proximal   toward elbow_

   C. Why? _to direct CR perpendicular to scaphoid_

13. Why is the entire PA hand sometimes routinely taken along with a lateral and oblique of individual dig
   its on a trauma patient when only a finger or thumb is ordered? _to rule out possible_
   secondary trauma to hand or wrist

14. For the carpal canal view (inferosuperior projection), how much should the CR be angled in relationship to the long axis of the hand? _____ 25-30° _____

15. If bilateral radiographs of the hands or wrists are ordered at the same time for possible trauma, should both hands or both wrists be placed side-by-side on the same film and taken with one exposure to reduce patient exposure?

    A. Yes or no? _____ yes _____

    B. If no, why not? _____

    C. If yes, why? _____ to reduce patient exposure _____

16. For possible trauma why is it important to take the lateral hand as a "fan" lateral rather than with

    all the fingers fully extended? _____ to demonstrate fingers individually _____

17. What are the basic projections for the following:

    A. Thumb _____ AP, oblique, lateral _____

    B. Fingers _____ PA   ob   lat _____

    C. Hand _____ PA   ob   lat _____

    D. Wrist _____ PA   ob   lat _____

18. What are the most common optional projections for the wrist? (List in order of most frequent use in U.S.)

    A. _____ ulnar flexion _____

    B. _____ carpal canal _____

    C. _____ radial flexion _____

    D. _____ carpal bridge _____

Review Exercise D   Positioning of Forearm, Elbow, Mid and Distal Humerus

Textbook: pp 130-144
Audio-visuals: Unit 5, slides 17-50

1. To use the anode-heel effect to the best advantage for an AP or lateral forearm, which should be placed at the cathode end of the x-ray beam, the elbow or the wrist? ___elbow___

2. What size film should be used for an adult AP and lateral forearm, and how should it be divided?

   A. Size ___10x14___ ___11x14 or 14x17___

   B. Divided ___half___

3. For an AP or lateral forearm, how much of the wrist and elbow should be included on the film?

   ___all___ ___min 1"___

4. List the correct CR location for the following:

   A. AP or lateral forearm ___midshaft___

   B. AP or oblique elbow ___elbow___

   C. Lateral elbow ___elbow___

5. What projections are required for a trauma elbow if the patient has elbow flexed about 90° with severe pain when attempting to extend elbow?

   A. ___AP forearm___   c. ___lateral elbow___

   B. ___AP humerus___

6. What specific anatomy is best shown on:

   A. Internal oblique elbow? ___coronoid process___

   B. External oblique elbow? ___radial head + neck___

7. The olecranon process of the elbow is best shown on what projection? ___lateral elbow___

8. The hand should be in what position for an internal oblique elbow? ___flat palm down___

9. Special trauma views of elbow:

   A. To better visualize the radial head, neck and tuberosity and the articular margin of capitulum, the elbow is flexed (a) ___90___ degrees, the hand is (b) ___pronated___ and the CR is angled (c) ___45___ degrees (d) ___toward shoulder___ (in which direction?)

   B. To better visualize the coronoid process and the articular margin of the trochlea, the elbow is flexed (a) ___80___ degrees from extended position, the hand is (b) ___pronated___ and the CR is angled (c) ___45___ degrees (d) ___away from shoulder___ (in which direction?)

10. For optimum uniform density (utilizing the anode-heel effect), what body part should be at the cathode end of the x-ray beam for an AP or lateral humerus? _____shoulder_____

11. For an AP and lateral of the entire humerus on an average or larger adult patient:

    A. What size film should be used? ___~~17×9~~___ ___14×17___

    B. Should a grid be used? ___~~no~~___ ___yes___

12. What two projections of the humerus should be taken if the patient has a possible fracture of the mid or distal third of humerus?

    A. ___AP___

    B. ___cross table lateral___

13. Post reduction check films of the forearm, wrist or elbow in a cast should always include (a)___2___ projections taken at (b)___90___ degrees from each other to check for part alignment in (c) ___two___ dimensions.

Review Exercise E   Laboratory Activity   Textbook: pp 112-144

Part of these exercises can be carried out effectively under very simulated conditions using a piece of paper and doing the positioning on yourself. However, part of the exercises need to be carried out using another person as a "patient" in a radiographic laboratory or a general diagnostic room in a radiology department. An x-ray tube with a collimator, lead shields and film markers should be available to simulate actual conditions with a patient as closely as possible (without the final step of making the exposure). Parts B and C can be carried out in any room where illuminators are available.

A.   **Positioning Exercise**

Practice the following until you can do each of them accurately and without hesitation. Place a check by each when you have achieved this.

__1. Practice positioning on yourself, all basic and optional projections for the thumb, each finger, hand, wrist and elbow.

__2. On another person, simulate taking all basic and optional projections of all parts of the upper limb. Include the following steps as described in the textbook and audio-visuals.

- Correct central ray placement and centering of part to film
- Accurate collimation
- Lead shielding for film and patient
- Appropriate size and type of film holder with correct markers
- Use of proper immobilizing devices when needed
- Approximate correct exposure factors.

__3. Simulate a routine wrist in a cast. Include all steps as described in Number 2 above. (Remember the type of film holder needed and the conversion rule for exposure factors.)

4. Simulate positioning of the elbow with the following conditions:

__   A. Elbow is flexed about 45° and cannot be extended without severe pain.

__   B. Two special trauma elbow projections for additional views of the areas of the radial head and the coronoid process of ulna.

Optional

__5. Using a sectional phantom, take several projections of the hand, wrist and forearm with correct exposure factors. Evaluate the radiograph for correct positioning and correct exposure factors.

B.   **Review of Anatomy**

Use radiographs provided by your instructor.

__1. Examine radiographs of the hand, wrist, forearm, elbow and humerus and identify all bones and parts of bones and all joints as described in this chapter of the textbook and/or audio-visuals.

C. Film Critique and Evaluation

Your instructor will provide various radiographs of the upper limb for these exercises. Some will be optimal quality radiographs meeting all or most of the evaluation criteria described for each projection in the textbook and/or audio-visuals. Others will be of less than optimal quality and several will be unacceptable, requiring a repeat exam. You should evaluate each radiograph as specified below.

Place a check by the following when completed.

___ 1. Critique each radiograph based on evaluation criteria provided for that projection in the textbook and/or audio-visuals. The following criteria guidelines can be used and checked as each radiograph is evaluated. (Additional checks can be placed to the left for each criteria guideline if more than six radiographs are evaluated.)

    Radiographs   Criteria Guidelines

    1 2 3 4 5 6

    __ __ __ __ __ __   a. Correct film size and correct orientation of part to film?

    __ __ __ __ __ __   b. Correct alignment and/or centering of part to film or portion of film being used?

    __ __ __ __ __ __   c. Correct collimation and CR location?

    __ __ __ __ __ __   d. Pertinent anatomy well visualized?

    __ __ __ __ __ __   e. Motion?

    __ __ __ __ __ __   f. Optimal exposure (density and/or contrast)?

    __ __ __ __ __ __   g. Patient ID information and markers?

___ 2. Based on acceptable variances to criteria factors, determine which of these radiographs are acceptable and which are unacceptable and should have been repeated.

Important: It is important that you have successfully carried out all of the exercises described above before taking the self-test and before going to your instructor for the chapter evaluation exam. If you neglect these exercises, you will not be able to meet all the objectives for this chapter and may not receive a passing grade for this course.

Answers to Review Exercise A

1. A. 14   B. 5   C. 8   D. 27

2. A. proximal phalanx   B. distal phalanx

3. Interphalangeal

4. A. First metacarpal
   B. First metacarpophalangeal joint
   C. Proximal phalanx of 1st digit
   D. Interphalangeal joint
   E. Middle phalanx of 2nd digit
   F. Distal phalanx of 3rd digit
   G. Distal interphalangeal joint
   H. Proximal interphalangeal joint
   I. Proximal phalanx of 5th digit
   J. 5th metacarpophalangeal joint
   K. 5th metacarpal
   L. Carpometacarpal joint

5. A. Scaphoid (navicular)
   B. Lunate (semilunar)
   C. Triquetrum (triangular or cuneiform)
   D. Pisiform
   E. Trapezium (greater multangular)
   F. Trapezoid (lesser multangular)
   G. Capitate (os magnum)
   H. Hamate (unciform)

6. Capitate (os magnum)

7. (a) hamate   (b) hamulus

8. Scaphoid (navicular)

9. A. Lunate
   B. Triquetrum
   C. Pisiform
   D. Hamulus of hamate
   E. Capitate
   F. Trapezoid
   G. Trapezium
   H. Scaphoid

   I. 1st metacarpal (thumb)
   J. Trapezium
   K. Trapezoid
   L. Capitate
   M. Hamulus of hamate
   N. Pisiform
   O. Triquetrum

If you missed more than 10 blanks, you should review this section again in the textbook and/or audio-visuals before continuing.

Answers to Review Exercise B

1. (a) Radius   (b) Ulna

2. A. Radial notch
    B. Coronoid tubercle
    C. Coronoid process
    D. Trochlear (semilunar) notch
    E. Olecranon process

3. A. Styloid process of radius
    B. Radius
    C. Shaft of radius
    D. Radial tuberosity
    E. Neck of radius
    F. Head of radius
    G. Shaft of ulna
    H. Ulna
    I. Ulnar notch
    J. Head of ulna
    K. Styloid process of ulna

4. Radius

5. Radius

6. Ulna

7. (a) Proximal radioulnar joint
    (b) Distal radioulnar joint

8. A. Radius
    B. Head of radius
    C. Capitulum (capitellum)
    D. Lateral epicondyle
    E. Radial fossa
    F. Coronoid fossa
    G. Medial epicondyle
    H. Condyle of humerus
    I. Trochlea
    J. Trochlear sulcus
    K. Ulna

9. (a) Capitulum
    (b) Capitellum

10. Medial

11. (a) Coronoid fossa,
    (b) Radial fossa,
    (c) Olecranon fossa

12. A. Trochlear sulcus
    B. Outer ridges of trochlea and capitulum
    C. Trochlear notch of ulna

13. (a) Ulnar flexion
    (b) Radial flexion

14. Radial deviation

15. Results in cross over (superimposition) of radius and ulna

16. A. Synovial
    B. Diarthrodial (freely movable)
    C. 1. Pivot
        2. Hinge
        3. Hinge
        4. Saddle
        5. Condyloid
        6. Saddle
        7. Gliding
        8. Gliding
        9. Condyloid

If you missed more than 11 blanks, you should review this section again in the textbook and/or audio-visuals before continuing.

Answers to Review Exercise C

1. A.   50-70
    B.   Shortest possible
    C.   Small
    D.   Minimum 40"
    E.   For body parts measuring over 10 cm.
    F.   Detail screen, table top (non-bucky)
    G.   5-7
    H.   (a) 8-10,   (b) double
    I.   3-4
    J.   (a) soft tissue margins
         (b) fine trabecular markings of
              all bones being radiographed

2. A.   Four-sided collimation should be used if
         the film size is large enough to prevent
         the cutting off of any essential anatomy.
    B.   Draw a large imaginary "x" from corner
         to corner, the exact center of which will
         indicate CR location.

3. Of reproductive age, (generally 50 and younger)

4. A.   1st MP joint
    B.   PIP joint
    C.   3rd MP joint
    D.   MP joint
    E.   Mid carpal area
    F.   To scaphoid, 3/4" proximal and
         3/4" lateral to 1st MP joint
    G.   1" distal to base of 3rd metacarpal
    H.   Midpoint of distal forearm about
         1.5" proximal to wrist joint

5. Thumb projected AP, finger PA

6. A.   Short exposure time
    B.   Immobilization

7. A.   None
    B.   Medial
    C.   Medial
    D.   Medial or lateral
    E.   Lateral
    F.   Lateral

8. To prevent motion while placing all digits
    parallel to film (to demonstrate open joint
    spaces without motion).

9. 4-5

10. 45 degrees

11. PA ulnar flexion (radial deviation)

12. A.   15-20°
    B.   Toward elbow
    C.   To direct CR perpendicular to scaphoid
         (prevents foreshortening)

13. To rule out possible secondary trauma or
    pathology to other aspects of the hand or
    wrist.

14. 25-30°

15. A.   No
    B.   The CR would be incorrectly placed.

16. To demonstrate fingers individually
    without superimposition.

17. A.   AP, oblique and lateral
    B.   PA, oblique and lateral
    C.   PA, oblique and lateral
    D.   PA, oblique and lateral

18. A.   Ulnar flexion
    B.   Carpal canal
    C.   Radial flexion
    D.   Carpal bridge

If you missed more than 10 blanks, you should review
this section again in the textbook and/or audio-visuals
before continuing.

Answers to Review Exercise D

1. Elbow

2. A.   11 x 14 or 14 x 17
   B.   In half lengthwise

3. Minimum of 1"

4. A.   Mid forearm
   B.   Mid elbow joint (which is about 3/4" distal to mid point of line connecting the epicondyles).
   C.   Mid elbow joint (which is about 1 1/2" medial to posterior surface of olecranon process).

5. A.   Lateral flexed 90°
   B.   2 APs, one with humerus parallel to film and one with forearm parallel.

6. A.   Coronoid process
   B.   Radial head and neck

7. Lateral elbow

8. Pronated or palm down

9. A.   (a) 90   (b) pronated   (c) 45   (d) toward the shoulder
   B.   (a) 80   (b) pronated   (c) 45   (d) away from the shoulder

10. Shoulder

11. A.   14 x 17
    B.   Yes

12. A.   AP without attempting to rotate arm
    B.   Crosstable lateral of mid and distal humerus without rotating arm

13. (a) Two   (b) 90   (c) two

If you missed more than 6 blanks, you should review this section again in the textbook and/or audio-visuals before continuing.

Self-Test

My score = _____ %

Directions: Take this self-test only after completing all the review exercises and laboratory activities in this chapter. Complete directions including grading requirements are described in the front pages of this workbook and in the self-test of Chapter 1.

Test

There are 100 blanks. Each correct blank is worth 1 point. (Spelling is important so correct any misspellings as you grade your test.)

1. Fill in the number of bones for the following:

    A. Phalanges   _14_

    B. Metacarpals   _5_

    C. Carpals   _8_ .

2. Fill in the correct terms for the following joints:

    A. Between the two bones of the first digit (thumb)
    IP 1st digit

    B. Between the first metacarpal and the proximal phalanx of the thumb
    MCP joint 1st digit

    C. Between the middle and distal phalanges of the 4th digit
    distal IP joint

    D. Between the carpals and the 1st metacarpal
    carpometacarpal

    E. Between the forearm and the carpals
    ~~radioulnat~~ RADIOCARPAL

3. Is the 1st metacarpal on the lateral or medial aspect of the hand? _~~medial~~ lateral_ ✓

4. List the carpals, include secondary names where indicated:

Proximal row, starting   A. _navicular_ (_scaphoid_)

from lateral side   B. _lunate_ (_semilunar_)

      C. _triangular_ (_triquetrum_)

      or

      (_cuneiform_)

      D. _pisiform_

Digital row, starting   E. _greater multangular_ (_trapezium_)

from lateral side   F. _lesser multangular_ (_trapezoid_)

      G. _capitate_ (_os magnum_)

      H. _hamate_ (_unciform_)

5. Which carpal contains a "hook-like" process? _hamate_ _unciform_

6. Which carpal articulates with the thumb? _trapezium_ _greater multangular_

7. Which carpal is most commonly fractured? _scaphoid / navicular_

8. A. What are two names for the special projection of the scaphoid?

   ulnar flexion or _radial deviation_

   B. How much and which direction is the CR angled for this projection? _15° -20° toward_

   the elbow   PROXIMAL

9. Which bone of the forearm articulates with the carpal bones? _radius_

10. Which three carpals are involved with the total wrist joint? A. _SCAPHOID_

   B. _LUNATE_   C. _TRIQUETRUM_

11. Indicate which of the bones of the forearm is lateral and which is medial:

   A. Lateral _radius_

   B. Medial _ulna_

12. What is the correct name for the depression on the lateral side of the coronoid process with which the head

of the radius articulates? _~~radial fossa~~_   RADIAL NOTCH

13. Indicate which bone of the forearm articulates most directly with the following:

A. Carpal bones _____ *radius* _____

B. Humerus _____ *ulna* _____

14. Identify the anatomy of this frontal view of the right radius and ulna as labeled:

A. _____ *styloid process* _____

B. _____ *radius* _____ (lateral bone of forearm)

C. _____ *shaft* _____

D. _____ *radial tuberosity* _____

E. _____ *neck* _____

F. _____ *head* _____

G. _____ ~~*radial tuberosity*~~ *CORONOID PROCESS* _____

H. _____ ~~*coronoid tuberosity*~~ *TROCHLEAR NOTCH* _____

I. _____ *olecranon process* _____

J. _____ *shaft* _____

K. _____ *ulna* _____ (medial bone of forearm)

L. _____ *ULNAR NOTCH (on radius)* _____

M. _____ *HEAD OF ULNA* _____

N. _____ *styloid process* _____

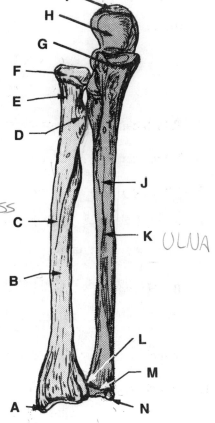

RADIUS

ULNA

Fig. 4-8

15. Identify the anatomy on this frontal view of the elbow:

   A. _CORONOID FOSSA_

   B. _medial epicondyle_

   C. _humeral condyle_

   D. _trochlea_

   E. _trochlear sulcus_

   F. _ulna_

   G. _radius_

   H. _head of radius_

   I. _capitullum_

   J. _lateral epicondyle_

   K. _radial fossa_

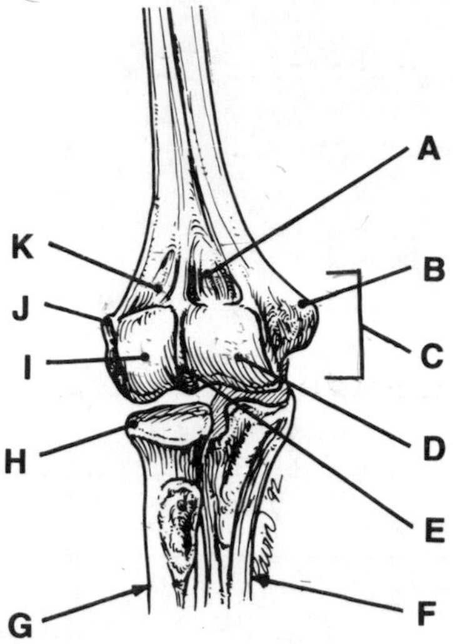

Fig. 4-9

16. The depressions on the anterior distal humerus are (a) _radial fossa_ and (b) _CORONOID fossa_

17. The depression on the posterior distal humerus is _olecranon fossa_

18. In what position should the hand be for the following?

   A. AP elbow _supine_

   B. Internal oblique elbow _pronated_

19. Why should a forearm never be taken as an AP projection? _the radius and ulna are crossed_

20. Which part of the elbow is best demonstrated on an internal oblique elbow? _olecranon CORONOID PROCESS_

21. Which part is best demonstrated on an external oblique elbow? _radial head & neck_

22. Which view best demonstrates the olecranon process? _Jones lateral elbow_

23. Joint classifications:

    A. Structural classification of all joints of upper limb? _____

    B. Mobility classification of all joints of upper limb? _____

    C. Movement type of first MP joint? _____

    D. Movement 2nd to 5th MP joint? _____

    E. Movement type of all IP joints? _____

    F. Movement type of wrist joint? _____

24. What are two ways motion can be avoided?

    A. _immobilization - sponges_

    B. _short exposure time_

25. Fill in the basic projections, size and type of film holder and the central ray location for the following exams:

	Basic Projections	Size & Type of Film Holder	Central Ray
A. 1st digit THUMB	(a) AP lat, obl	(b) 9×9 extr. 8×10 or 10×12	(c) MCP joint
B. 4th digit	(a) PA lat obl	(b) 9×9 extr. 8×10	(c) prox IP joint
C. Hand	(a) PA lat obl	(b) 9×9 8×10 or 10×12 10×12	(c) 3rd MCP
D. Wrist	(a) PA lat obl	(b) 9×9 8×10	(c) mid carpal
E. Wrist and forearm in cast	(a) PA lat	(b) 10×12 extr.	(c) midwrist
F. Elbow ✗	(a) AP lat obl	(b) 14×17 10×12 extr.	(c) elbow

26. Describe the criteria for evaluating a true lateral elbow. _90° angle, 3 rings_

    _____

    _____

27. Grids are commonly used for parts measuring over _10 cm_.

28. How much should exposure factors be increased for:

    A.   Small to medium dry plaster cast? _5-7_____ kVp

    B.   Large or wet plaster cast? _8-10___ kVp or __2x___ mAs

    C.   Average fiberglass cast? _3-4___ kVp

29. How much should kVp be increased from a PA hand to a lateral hand? _4-5____

Answers to Self-Test

1. A.   14
   B.   5
   C.   8

2. A.   Interphalangeal joint of first digit
   B.   1st metacarpophalangeal joint
   C.   Distal interphalangeal joint of 4th digit
   D.   1st carpometacarpal joint
   E.   Radiocarpal joint

3. Lateral (remember this assumes the anatomical position)

4. A.   Scaphoid (navicular)
   B.   Lunate (semilunar)
   C.   Triquetrum (triangular or cuneiform)
   D.   Pisiform
   E.   Trapezium (greater multangular)
   F.   Trapezoid (lesser multangular)
   G.   Capitate (os magnum)
   H.   Hamate (unciform)

5. Hamate

6. Trapezium

7. Scaphoid

8. A.   Ulnar flexion or radial deviation
   B.   15-20°, proximal or toward elbow

9. Radius

10. A.   Scaphoid
    B.   Lunate
    C.   Triquetrum

11. A.   Radius
    B.   Ulna

12. Radial notch

13. A.   Radius
    B.   Ulna

14. A.   Styloid process of radius
    B.   Radius
    C.   Shaft
    D.   Radial tuberosity
    E.   Neck of radius
    F.   Radial head
    G.   Coronoid process
    H.   Trochlear (semilunar) notch
    I.   Olecranon process
    J.   Shaft
    K.   Ulna
    L.   Ulnar notch
    M.   Head of ulna
    N.   Styloid process of ulna

15. A.   Coronoid fossa
    B.   Medial epicondyle
    C.   Humeral condyle
    D.   Trochlea
    E.   Trochlear sulcus
    F.   Ulna
    G.   Radius
    H.   Head of radius
    I.   Capitulum
    J.   Lateral epicondyle
    K.   Radial fossa

16. (a)   the coronoid fossa
    (b)   the radial fossa

17. the olecranon fossa

18. A.   Supinated
    B.   Pronated

19. The radius crosses over and superimposes the ulna.

20. Coronoid process

21. Radial head and neck

22. Lateral elbow

23. A.   Synovial
    B.   Diarthrodial (freely movable)
    C.   Saddle
    D.   Condyloid
    E.   Hinge
    F.   Condyloid

24. A.   Immobilization
    B.   Short exposure times

25. A.   (a)   AP, lat., obli.
        (b)   8 x 10 or 10 x 12, detail screen
        (c)   1st MP joint

    B.   (a)   PA, obli., lat.
         (b)   8 x 10, detail screen
         (c)   Proximal IP joint

    C.   (a)   PA, obli., lat.
         (b)   8 x 10 or 10 x 12 detail screen
         (c)   3rd MP joint

    D.   (a)   PA, obli., lat.
         (b)   8 x 10 detail
         (c)   Midwrist

    E.   (a)   PA and lat.
         (b)   10 x 12 detail
         (c)   Mid point of film

Answers to Self-Test continued

25. *(continued)*

    F. (a)　AP, obli., lat
       (b)　10 x 12 detail
       (c)　Mid elbow joint

26. Appearance of 3 concentric or uniform
    arcs, (1) the trochlear sulcus, (2) medial
    ridges of trochlea and capitulum and
    (3) the trochlear notch

27. 10 cm.

28. A. 5 to 7
    B. 8 to 10 or double
    C. 3 or 4

29. 4 to 5 kVp

Chapter 5
Proximal Humerus and Shoulder Girdle

Rationale

Radiographic examinations of the shoulder girdle including the routine shoulder, the clavicle, and the upper scapula are among the more difficult and most challenging of any examination involving the upper limbs. The shape and general structure of the shoulder girdle is such that specific projections involving angles and certain rotations are required to visualize these structures on x-ray film. This requires a good understanding of the anatomy and the relative positions of anatomical structures of the bones of the shoulder girdle.

You will need to understand what basic projections should be taken for each examination involving the proximal humerus and the shoulder girdle and know which structures are best demonstrated on each projection.

Specific positioning exercises are described in your workbook which will guide you in positioning for each exam as described in this chapter. The film critique exercises will help you learn to critique and to judge radiographs to determine how they can be improved. You will also learn how to evaluate as to whether they are of acceptable diagnostic quality or if they need to be repeated and improved.

Successful completion of all the exercises in this chapter should provide you with enough knowledge and skill to perform actual radiographic examinations on patients under the supervision of a technologist.

Chapter Objectives

After you have successfully completed all the activities of this chapter, you will be able, with at least 80% accuracy, to: (applicable to a written and/or oral examination and demonstration)

___ 1. Identify, both on drawings and radiographs, all anatomy of the proximal humerus and the shoulder girdle as described in the textbook and/or audio-visuals.

___ 2. Describe relative positions or locations of prominent structures involving the proximal humerus and the shoulder girdle as described in the textbook and/or audio-visuals.

___ 3. List and describe basic and optional projections, the type and size of film holder, the central ray location with correct angles and the structures best demonstrated on each projection.

___ 4. Position on a model or a phantom all basic and optional projections described in the textbook and/or audio-visuals.

___ 5. Critique and evaluate each radiograph according to evaluation criteria described in the textbook and/or audio-visuals.

Given several radiographs of the proximal humerus, shoulder, clavicle, and scapula to view:

___ 6. Discriminate between radiographs which are acceptable and those which are unacceptable due to exposure factors, collimation, or overall lack of positioning accuracy.

Prerequisite

The only prerequisite knowledge requirement for this chapter is an understanding of radiographic terminology and the principles of exposure, radiation protection and positioning as described in Chapter 1. It is strongly suggested that a mandatory prerequisite for this chapter be the successful completion of Chapter 1.

Recommended Supplementary References

The following supplementary references, which are described in more detail in Chapter 1, are listed in a suggested order of importance and value to understanding this material.

1. *Merrill's ...*, Vol 1, pp 111-159

2. *Clark's ...*, pp 69-88

3. *Eisenberg ...*, pp 75-94

Review Exercise A Proximal Humerus and Shoulder Girdle 5

Learning Exercises

The following review exercises should be completed only after careful study of the associated pages in the textbook and/or audio-visuals as indicated by each exercise.

After completing each of these individual exercises, check your answers with the answer sheets which follow before continuing to the next exercise.

Part I. RADIOGRAPHIC ANATOMY

Review Exercise A Anatomy of Proximal Humerus, Clavicle and Scapula

Textbook: pp 145-150
Audio-visuals, Unit 6, slides 19-32

1. Identify the parts of the proximal humerus shown with neutral rotation of the arm which results in an oblique position of the proximal humerus.

   A. surgical neck
   B. intertubercular groove (BICIPITAL GROOVE)
   C. greater tubercle tuberosity
   D. head
   E. anatomical neck
   F. lesser tubercle tuberosity
   G. shaft body

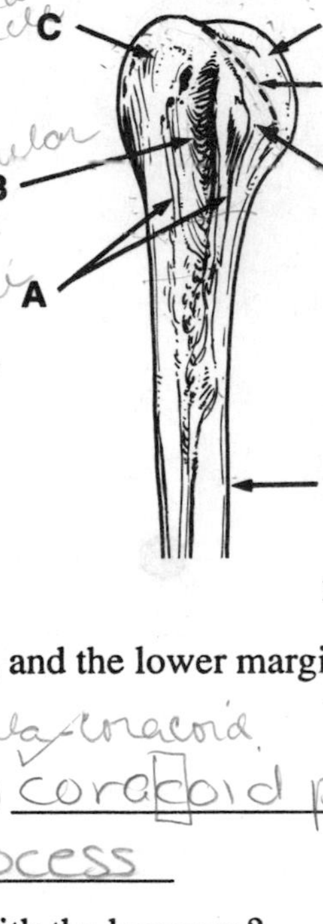

Fig. 5-1

2. The upper margin of the scapula is at the level of the (a) 2nd rib, and the lower margin at the (b) 7th rib.
3. Which portion of the upper scapula is located most anteriorly? (a) coracoid process most posteriorly? (b) ~~Spine~~ acromion process
4. What is the name of the portion of the scapula which articulates with the humerus? glenoid cavity (fossa)
5. The costal surface of the scapula refers to the anterior (ventral) surface.
6. What is the name of the joint connecting the scapula and clavicle? acromioclavicular
7. What are the three main parts of the clavicle? (a) acromial end, (b) sternal end and (c) shaft. Which extremity is more triangular in shape? (d) sternal

8. What is the anatomical name for the armpit? _____axilla_____

9. What is the name of the very prominent structure visible on the posterior scapula which adds strength to the body of the scapula? _____spine_____

10. What are the names of the two fossae located on the posterior scapula?

    A. _____infraspinous_____

    B. _____supraspinous_____

11. Fill in the correct (a) structural classification, (b) mobility classification and (c) movement type for the following:

    A. Shoulder joint   (a) _____synovial_____ (b) _____diarthrosis_____ (c) _____ball + socket_____

    B. Sternoclavicular joint   (a) _____synovial_____ (b) _____diarthrosis_____ (c) _____gliding_____

    C. Acromioclavicular joint   (a) _____synovial_____ (b) _____diarthrosis_____ (c) _____gliding_____

    D. Epiphyses of humerus   (a) _____cartilaginous_____ (b) _____synarthrosis_____ (c) _____—_____
    (on a child)

    1) ball + socket   3) gliding   5) condyloid
    synovial — 2) hinge   4) pivot   6) saddle
    fibrous — suture + syndesmoses
    cartilagenous → symphysis · synchondroses

12. Fill in the following from frontal and lateral drawings of the scapula:

    A. _____glenoid cavity_____

    B. _____acromion_____

    C. _____coracoid process_____

    D. _____scapular notch_____

    E. _____superior border_____

    F. _____superior angle_____

    G. _____medial border_____

    H. _____inferior angle_____

    I. _____lateral border_____

    J. _____neck_____

    K. _____lateral angle (head)_____

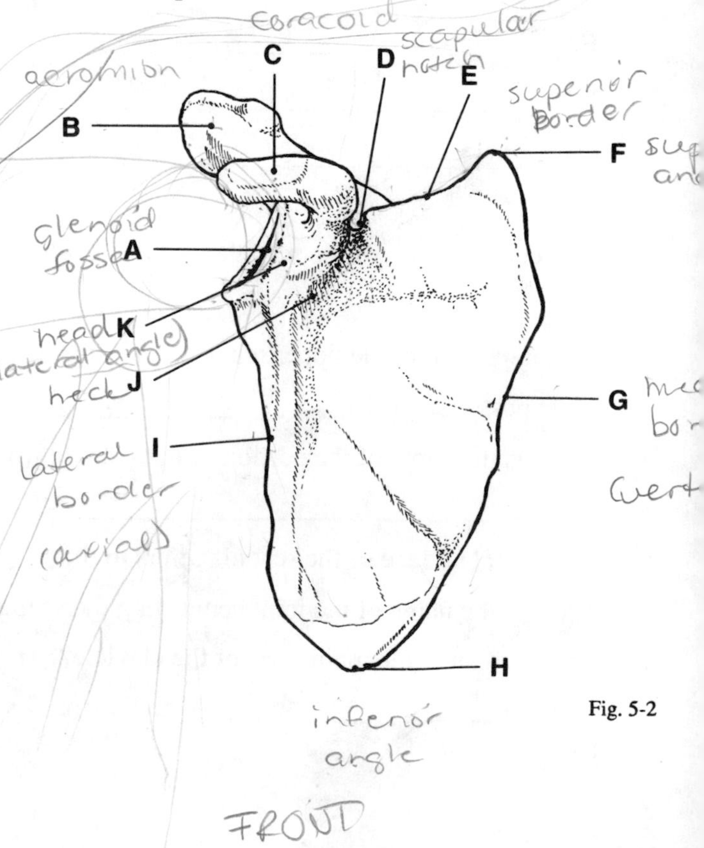

Fig. 5-2

12. *(continued)*

✓ L. <u>acromion</u>

✓ M. <u>coracoid process</u>

✓ N. <u>glenoid cavity</u>

O. <u>body ventral surface</u>

P. <u>inferior angle</u>

Q. <u>dorsal surface</u>

R. <u>ventral surface body</u>

S. <u>spine of scapula</u>

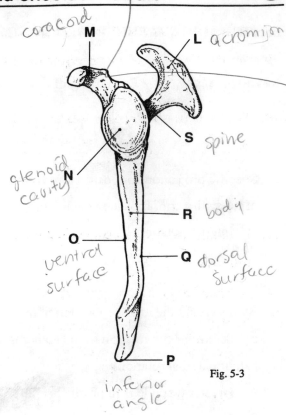

coracoid

M

L acromion

glenoid cavity

N

S spine

O

ventral surface

R body

Q dorsal surface

P

inferior angle

Fig. 5-3

Part II. RADIOGRAPHIC POSITIONING

Review Exercise B   Positioning of Proximal Humerus, Shoulder, Scapula and Clavicle

Textbook: pp 151-167
Audio-visuals, Unit 6, slides 33-61

1. Specific projections or positions of the proximal humerus and shoulder can be obtained by rotation of the entire arm. Indicate which projection /position (AP, oblique, or lateral) is obtained by:

   A. Internal rotation ___lateral___

   B. External rotation ___AP___

   C. Neutral rotation ___oblique___

2. By observing the relative location of the greater tubercle of the proximal humerus on the radiograph, one can determine the rotation of the humerus. Indicate the correct rotation for the following: (neutral, internal, or external rotation)

   A. Greater tubercle is in profile laterally ___ex ro___

   B. Greater tubercle is located anteriorly and medially ___in ro___

   C. Greater tubercle is located anteriorly and laterally ___neutral___

3. What are the basic projections for a shoulder exam if the patient's history does not indicate a possible fracture? ___AP in ro ex ro axilla___

4. What projections should be taken for the proximal humerus with a possible dislocation or fracture?
   ___AP transthoracic lateral___

5. Where is the correct central ray location on a shoulder examination? ___coracoid process___

6. As you position a patient for a shoulder exam, by viewing the patient's arm and elbow how can you determine if the arm is rotated sufficiently for: _elbow_

   A. An internal rotation shoulder? ___epicondyles perpendicular to film___

   B. An external rotation shoulder? ___epicondyles parallel to film___

7. Which angle and approximately how many degrees should be used on:

   A. PA clavicle ___caudal___ angle, ___5° - 15°___ degrees

   B. AP clavicle ___cephalic___ angle, ___10° - 20°___ degrees

8. A thin-shouldered patient will require **more** or less angle for a clavicle projection than a large-shouldered patient? ___more___

9. Should a scapula exam on a patient with severe pain to this area be taken **supine** or **erect** if the patient is able? ___erect___

10. The clavicle projection on a patient with severe kyphosis of the spine should be taken **AP** or **PA**? _PA_

11. Complete the following for an acromioclavicular joint exam:

    A. Basic projections ___AP bilateral -one w/weights one w/o wts.___

    B. SID ___72"___

    C. Taken erect or supine ___erect___

12. True or False: (explain why)

    For the AP projection of the acromioclavicular joints with weights, it is best to have the patient firmly hold onto the weights with each hand. ___should be tied ,so arms + ___ ___shoulders can be relaxed___

13. The apical oblique projection is frequently taken for possible shoulder dislocation, glenoid fracture or Hill-Sachs lesions. Describe the correct patient position and central ray angle for this projection.

    A. Patient position: ___supine erect 45° posterior obl, side of___

    B. Central ray angle: ___horizontal 45° caudal___ ___interest against film___

14. For the apical oblique projection, a **posterior** dislocation of the humerus will project the humerus **superior** or **inferior** to the glenoid cavity (a) ___superior___ , and an **anterior** dislocation will project it **inferior** or **superior**? (b) ___inferior___

15. True or False. (explain why)

    The inferosuperior axial projection is a good projection for determining a possible dislocation of the shoulder. ___false   could cause further dislocation___

16. List the basic projections, correct size, type of film holder, and the correct placement position of the film for the following:

	Basic Projections (a)	Film Size - 8 x 10 - 10 x 12 - 7 x 17 - 14 x 17 (b)	Film Holder - screen (non-grid) - bucky (grid) (c)	Placement - crosswise - lengthwise (d)
A. Scapula	AP lat	10×12	bucky	lengthwise
B. Clavicle	AP	10×12	bucky	crosswise
C. Shoulder (trauma)	AP trans, lateral	10×12	screen	crosswise
D. AC joints (average or small patient)	w/wo (2) AP bilat	7×17 14×17	screen	crosswise
E. AC joints (large, broad patient)	w-wo (2) AP bilat	2 8×10s	grid	crosswise
F. Shoulder (non-trauma)	AP in ro ex ro	10×12	grid	crosswise

17. Indicate which drawing demonstrates an **internal** and which an **external** rotation of the humerus.

A. external ___   B. internal ___
     AP   lateral

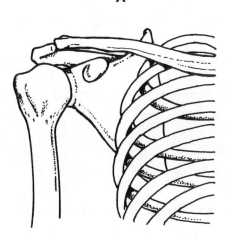

A

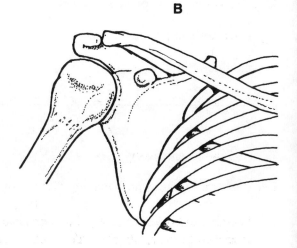

B

Fig. 5-4

Review Exercise C   Laboratory Activity   Textbook: pp 155-167

This part of the learning activity exercise series needs to be carried out in a radiographic laboratory or a general diagnostic room in a radiology department. Part B can be carried out in a classroom or any room where illuminators are available.

A. Positioning Exercise

For this section you need another person to act as your "patient." Practice the following until you can do each of them accurately and without hesitation. It is important to achieve both accuracy and speed in radiographic positioning. Place a check by each when you have achieved this.

Include the following details as you simulate the basic projections for each exam listed below:

- patient shielding as needed
- correct size and type of film holder
- correct location of central ray and correct centering of part to film
- correct placement of markers
- accurate collimation
- proper use of immobilizing devices
- approximate correct exposure factors
- correct instructions to your "patient" as you "make" the exposure

___ 1. Shoulder exam (no indication of fracture to humerus)

___ 2. Clavicle

___ 3. Scapula

___ 4. AC (acromioclavicular) joints

Optional: Using either a sectional or fully articulated phantom, produce a diagnostic radiograph for each of the following:

___ 1. AP shoulder

___ 2. AP clavicle

___ 3. AP scapula

B. Review of Anatomy

Use those radiographs provided by your instructor.

1. Examine radiographs of the shoulder, scapula and clavicle and identify all anatomical parts as described in the textbook and/or audiovisuals.

C. Film Critique and Evaluation

Your instructor will provide radiographs of the shoulder, clavicle and scapula for these exercises. Some will be of optimal quality meeting all or nearly all evaluation criteria as described in the textbook and/or audio-visuals. Others will be less than optimal, and several will be unacceptable requiring repeat exams. You should critique or evaluate each radiograph carefully and individually following the steps below.

___ 1.   Critique each radiograph based on evaluation criteria provided for each projection in the textbook and/or audio-visuals. The following criteria guidelines can be used and checked as each radiograph is evaluated.

Radiographs   Criteria Guidelines

1   2   3   4   5   6

__ __ __ __ __ __   a. Correct film size and correct orientation of part to film?

__ __ __ __ __ __   b. Correct alignment and/or centering of part to film or portion of film being used?

__ __ __ __ __ __   c. Correct collimation and CR location?

__ __ __ __ __ __   d. Pertinent anatomy well visualized?

__ __ __ __ __ __   e. Motion?

__ __ __ __ __ __   f. Optimal exposure (density and/or contrast)?

__ __ __ __ __ __   g. Patient ID information and markers?

___ 2.   Based on acceptable variances to criteria factors, determine which of these radiographs are acceptable and which are unacceptable and should have been repeated.

Important: It is important that you have successfully carried out all of the exercises described above before taking the self-test and before going to your instructor for the chapter evaluation exam. If you neglect these exercises, you will not be able to meet all the objectives for this chapter and may not receive a passing grade for this course.

Answers to Review Exercise A

1. A. Surgical neck
   B. Intertubercular (bicipital) groove
   C. Greater tubercle (tuberosity)
   D. Head
   E. Anatomical neck
   F. Lesser tubercle (tuberosity)
   G. Shaft (body)

2. (a) 2nd   (b) 7th

3. (a) coracoid process   (b) acromion process

4. Glenoid cavity (fossa)

5. Ventral or anterior

6. Acromioclavicular (AC) joint

7. (a) shaft (b) sternal extremity (c) acromial extremity (d) sternal

8. Axilla

9. Spine of scapula

10. A. supraspinatus fossa
    B. infraspinatus fossa

11. A. (a) Synovial   (b) Diarthrosis   (c) Ball and socket
    B. (a) Synovial   (b) Diarthrosis   (c) Gliding
    C. (a) Synovial   (b) Diarthrosis   (c) Gliding
    D. (a) Cartilaginous   (b) Synarthrosis   (c) —

12. A. Glenoid cavity (fossa)
    B. Acromion process
    C. Coracoid process
    D. Scapular notch
    E. Superior border
    F. Superior angle
    G. Medial (vertebral) border
    H. Inferior angle
    I. Lateral (axillary) border
    J. Neck
    K. Lateral angle (head)

    L. Acromion process
    M. Coracoid process
    N. Glenoid cavity (fossa)
    O. Ventral (costal or anterior) surface
    P. Inferior angle
    Q. Dorsal (posterior) surface
    R. Body of scapula
    S. Spine of scapula

If you missed more than 9 blanks, you should review this section again in the textbook and/or audio-visuals before continuing.

Answers to Review Exercise B

1. A. Lateral
   B. AP
   C. Oblique

2. A. External rotation
   B. Internal rotation
   C. Neutral rotation

3. AP internal rotation and AP external rotation

4. AP and transthoracic lateral or scapular Y

5. Coracoid process

6. A. Epicondyles should be perpendicular to plane of film
   B. Epicondyles should be parallel to plane of film

7. A. Caudal, 5-15 degrees
   B. Cephalic, 10-20 degrees

8. More

9. Erect (less painful if patient can stand or be seated erect)

10. PA

11. A. Two AP's, bilateral, one with weights and one without weights
    B. 72 inches
    C. Erect

12. False (The weights should be tied to the wrists so the hands, arms and shoulders can be relaxed to determine possible AC separation.)

13. A. Erect, 45° posterior oblique, side of interest against film.
    B. 45° caudal

14. (a) superiorly   (b) inferiorly

15. False (This projection should never be attempted if a fracture or dislocation is suspected because it could result in more dislocation of fracture.)

16. A. (a) AP, lateral,   (b) 10 x 12,   (c) bucky or grid,   (d) lengthwise
    B. (a) AP,   (b) 10 x 12,   (c) bucky or grid,   (d) crosswise
    C. (a) AP, transthoracic lateral, or scapular Y,   (b) 10 x 12,   (c) screens,   (d) crosswise
    D. (a) AP bilateral with and without weights,   (b) 14 x 17 or 7 x 17,   (c) screens,   (d) crosswise
    E. (a) AP bilateral with and without weights,   (b) two 8 x 10s,   (c) grid,   (d) crosswise
    F. (a) AP internal and external rotation,   (b) 10 x 12s,   (c) grid,   (d) crosswise

17. A. External
    B. Internal

If you missed more than 11 blanks, you should review this section again in the textbook and/or audio-visuals before continuing.

Self-Test

My score = _____ %

Directions: Take this self-test only after completing all the review exercises and laboratory activities in this chapter. Complete directions including grading requirements are described in the front pages of this workbook and in the self-test of Chapter 1.

Test

There are 50 blanks. Each correct blank is worth 2 points. (Spelling is important so correct any misspellings as you grade your test.)

1. What are two other terms which can be used to describe the <u>ventral</u> surface of the scapula?

   A. _costal_   ✓   dorsal-
   posterior
   B. _anterior_

2. What is the correct term for the armpit? _axilla_ ✓

3. The upper margin of the scapula is at the level of the (a) _2nd_ ✓ rib and the lower
   margin at the (b) _7th_ ✓ rib.

4. What is the primary function of the shoulder girdle? _connect the arm to_
   the body

5. What is the name of the joint connecting the two bones of the shoulder girdle? _acromioclavicular_ ✓

6. List the three borders of the scapula:

   A. _superior_ ✓
   B. _lateral (axillary)_ ✓
   C. _medial (vertebral)_ ✓

   Fill in the correct term describing the following areas or parts of the scapula:

   D. The most anterior process _coracoid_ ✓   acromion-posterior
   E. The part which articulates with the humerus _glenoid fossa_ ✓
   F. The structure separating the two posterior fossae _spine_ ✓
   Infraspinous
   supraspinous

6.   *(continued)*

G.   The notch on the superior border ___scapular notch___

H.   The expanded lateral portion of the spine ___ACROMION___

I.   The process extending anteriorly to the glenoid fossa ___coracoid___

7.   The correct central ray location for an AP shoulder is to the ___coracoid process___.

8.   The basic projection(s) for the scapula is (are) ___AP lateral (y-view)___.

9.   A.   The correct term describing the area of the scapula where the vertebral and superior borders meet is ___neck SUPERIOR ANGLE___.

B.   Where do the axillary and superior borders meet? ___NECK LATERAL ANGLE (HEAD)___

C.   Where do the axillary and vertebral borders meet? ___INFERIOR ANGLE___

D.   The correct terms describing the two prominent fossae on the posterior scapula are___ ___infraspinous___ and ___supraspinous___.

10.   Write in true or false for the following statements. If the statement is false, write in the correct word(s) to make it true.

A.   The clavicle is usually shorter and less curved on females than males. ___T___

B.   The acromion process extends superiorly and anteriorly to the glenoid fossa.___F___ ___superior + posterior___   coracoid process is anter~

C.   For an AP projection of the clavicle, a 10 to 20 degree caudal angle should be used. ___F___ ___cephalic___   PA caudal

D.   More angle should be used on an AP clavicle for a thin patient. ___T___

E.   The coracoid process extends anteriorly to the glenoid fossa. ___T___

F.   The acromial extremity of the clavicle is more triangular in shape. ___F___ ___sternal___
     end

G.   The clavicle is a long bone with a double curvature with three main parts. ___T___

10. *(continued)*

H.   The film holders for a routine AP shoulder are two 10 x 12's placed lengthwise. ___F___

_____CROSSWISE_____

I.   Placing the epicondyles of the humerus perpendicular to the plane of the film will result in a good

internal rotation view of the shoulder. ___F___ *parallel*   *T, ex-ro*

perpendicular = ex ro   *parallel*

J.   A 72 inch SID should be used for an exam of the AC joints. ___T___

_____

K.   Synarthrosis refers to an immovable joint. ___T___ _amphiorthrosis - some_

movement

diarthrosis- freely moving

L.   A gliding type joint is classified as amphiarthrodial. ___F___ _diarthrosis_

_____

M.   The glenohumeral joint is a synovial, diarthrodial joint with a hinge movement type. ___F___

ball + socket

N.   Both the sternoclavicular and acromioclavicular joints are synovial, diarthrodial types, both with

gliding movements. ___T___

O.   All three joints of the shoulder girdle are enclosed in an articular capsule containing synovial fluid.

___T___

P.   The clavicle on a patient with kyphosis of the spine should be taken as an AP projection.

___F___ _PA_   _caudal angle_

Q.   The acromioclavicular joint projections should be taken erect rather than supine if patient's condition

allows. ___T___

11. The basic projections for a shoulder exam:

A.   With a possible fracture to the proximal humerus: ___AP lateral___ _transthoracic_ _lateral_

_____

B.   With no symptoms of a fracture or dislocation: ___AP inro ex ro___

axila

12. Which rotation will best demonstrate the greater tubercle of the humerus? (Internal or external)

    external ✓

13. Which rotation will result in a view of the proximal humerus in a near lateral position? _external AP_

    ~~external~~ _internal_

14. A. Which angle is required to project the clavicle above the scapula and rib on a (PA) projection?

    caudal

    B. On an AP projection? _10°-20°_ _cephalic_

15. What is the name of the joint connecting the shoulder girdle to the trunk? _sternoclavicular_

16. The two parts which form the upper "arms" of the "Y" on a lateral scapula position are the

    (a) _acromion_ and (b) _coracoid process_ , and

    the bottom "leg" is made up of the (c) _body_ .

Answers to Self-Test

1. A. Costal
   B. Anterior

2. Axilla

3. (a) 2nd (b) 7th

4. Connect upper limb to trunk

5. Acromioclavicular joint

6. A. medial (vertebral)
   B. superior
   C. lateral (axillary)

   D. Coracoid process
   E. Glenoid cavity (fossa)
   F. Spine ofscapula
   G. Scapular notch
   H. Acromion
   I. Coracoid process

7. Coracoid process

8. AP and lateral

9. A. Superior angle
   B. Lateral angle or head of scapula
   C. Inferior angle
   D. Supraspinatus and infraspinatus

10. A. True
    B. False, posteriorly & superiorly
    C. False, cephalic
    D. True
    E. True
    F. False, sternal extremity
    G. True
    H. False, crosswise
    I. True
    J. True
    K. True
    L. False, diarthrodial
    M. False, ball and socket movement
    N. True
    O. True
    P. False, PA
    Q. True

11. A. AP & transthoracic lateral
       or scapular Y
    B. AP with internal & external rotation

12. External

13. Internal

14. A. Caudal
    B. Cephalic

15. Sternoclavicular

16. (a) acromion
    (b) coracoid process
    (c) body of scapula

Chapter 6
Lower Limb

Foot, Ankle, Leg, Knee and Mid and Distal Femur

Rationale

If you wish to achieve accuracy and consistency and become a professional technologist, it is important that you learn the anatomy and the anatomical relationships of the lower limbs well so you will understand WHY certain specific projections are required to visualize each anatomical part on x-ray film. It is relatively easy to memorize certain basic projections and make radiographs of these parts but a good radiographer will be able to make necessary adjustments and will be able to modify certain projections to better demonstrate certain anatomical parts as requested by the physician or as indicated by the patient's clinical history.

A good technologist will also understand the importance of utilizing the central ray to the best advantage to "open up" certain joint spaces and to prevent distortion of anatomical parts which could prevent visualization of certain fractures or other pathology.

With the ever increasing awareness of the potential hazards to the public through medical uses of radiation, it is becoming more and more important that a technologist reach a level of competence that will minimize or eliminate entirely unnecessary exposure to patients through repeats, etc. A good understanding of anatomy and positioning of the foot and ankle as described in this chapter will help you reach this level of competence.

The limbs are sometimes considered some of the easier parts to radiograph but this is not necessarily true because the shape and positions of the bones at the ankle and knee joints and the many small bones of the foot result in much superimposition which make them very difficult to visualize on radiographs.

You must be able to critique the radiographs you have taken to know what errors you have made and know how these errors can be corrected. You must also know which anatomical parts need to be visualized on each radiograph and be able to critique films to see if these parts are all visualized well. You will learn how to evaluate radiographs for accuracy of positioning and exposure factors utilizing specific evaluation criteria.

Successful completion of all the exercises in this chapter should provide you with enough knowledge and skill to perform actual radiographic examinations of the lower limb on patients under the supervision of a technologist.

Chapter Objectives

After you have completed **all** the activities of this unit, you will be able, with at least 80% accuracy, to: (applicable to a written and/or oral examination and demonstration)

___ 1. Identify, both on drawings and radiographs, all anatomy of the foot, ankle, leg, knee, patella and femur as described in the textbook and/or audio-visuals.

___ 2. Identify joints and anatomical relationships of the foot, ankle, and knee as described in the textbook and/or audio-visuals.

___ 3. List both the preferred names and the secondary names for the tarsals as indicated in the textbook and/or audio-visuals.

___ 4. Identify all joints of the foot, ankle, leg and knee as to the correct classification and movement type.

___ 5. List two terms for describing the different projections taken for the foot and the terms describing the surface marking of the foot.

___ 6. List all basic and optional projections, and orientation of the film holder and the central ray locations and/or angles for the **toes, foot, ankle, os calcis, knee, patella, intercondyloid fossa and femur,** as described in the textbook and/or audiovisuals.

___ 7. List the basic projections for the foot, ankle, leg, knee or femur in a cast and describe the conversion rule for converting exposure factors from a routine non-cast limb to a cast.

___ 8. Position on a phantom or a model all basic and optional projections of the anatomical parts listed in Objective Number 6.

___ 9. Given the necessary equipment and a simulated patient (articulated phantom), produce a diagnostic radiograph for each basic projection of the foot, os calcis and ankle.

___ 10. Critique each radiograph based on evaluation criteria provided in the textbook and/or audio-visuals.

___ 11. Discriminate between those radiographs which are acceptable and those which are unacceptable because of exposure factors, collimation or positioning errors.

Prerequisite

The prerequisite knowledge requirement for this chapter is an understanding of radiographic terminology and the principles of exposure, radiation protection and positioning as described in Chapter 1. It is strongly suggested that a mandatory prerequisite for this chapter be the successful completion of Chapter 1.

Recommended Supplementary References

The following supplementary references, which are described in more detail in Chapter 1, are listed in a suggested order of importance and value to understanding this material.

1. *Merrill's ...,* Vol 1, pp 161-239

2. *Clark's ...,* pp 89-122

3. *Eisenberg ...,* pp 95-135

Learning Exercises

The following review exercises should be completed only after careful study of the associated pages in the textbook and/or audio-visuals as indicated by each exercise.

After completing each of these individual exercises, check your answers with the answer sheets which follow before continuing to the next exercise.

Part I. RADIOGRAPHIC ANATOMY

Review Exercise A Anatomy of Foot and Ankle   Textbook: pp 169-175
                                        Audio-visuals: Unit 7, slides 1-26

1. Fill in the number of bones for the following:

   A. Phalanges   _14_

   B. Metatarsal   _5_

   C. Tarsals   _7_   *hand has 8 carpals*

   D. Total   _26_

2. Name the parts (phalanges) of the following digits of the foot:

   A. 1st digit _proximal   distal_

   B. 2nd to 5th digits _proximal middle distal_

3. Name the correct joint(s) for the following: (List both the complete name and the initials)

   A. Between the phalanges of the 1st digit _IP   interphalangeal_

   B. Between the phalanges of the 5th digit _PIP   DIP   proximal distal_

   C. Between the talus and the calcaneus _TALOCALCANEAL (SUBTALAR)_

   D. Between the talus and the lower leg _ANKLE_

4. A. What are the bones forming the instep? _METATARSALS_

   B. Does the numbering start medially or laterally? _medial_

5. Name the three parts of each metatarsal:

   A. Proximal end _base_

   B. Mid _shaft_

   C. Distal end _head_

6. A. How many facets or articular surfaces are present in the talocalcaneal joint? _*subtalar*_ _3_

   B. The opening or space at this joint through which certain ligaments pass is called the _____
   TARSAL SINUS .

7. Fill in the correct term for the following tarsals: (Give secondary terms where applicable)

    A. Largest tarsal _____ calcaneus _____ OS CALCIS _____

    B. Second largest tarsal _____ talus _____ ASTRAGALUS _____

    C. Most posterior tarsal _____ calcaneus _____ OS CALCUS _____

    D. Most superior tarsal _____ TALUS _____ ASTRAGALUS _____

    E. Located between talus and cuneiforms _____ navicular _____ SCAPHOID

    F. Correct tarsal articulating distally with the following metatarsals:

       (1)   1st metatarsal _1ST CUNEIFORM_____

       (2)   2nd metatarsal _2ND CUNEIFORM_____

       (3)   3rd metatarsal _3RD CUNEIFORM_____

       (4)   4th metatarsal _CUBOID_____

       (5)   5th metatarsal _CUBOID_____

8. List all three bones making up the ankle joint: A. _TALUS_____, B. _TIBIA_____,

    C. _FIBULA_____.

9. Which bone of the distal leg is the smaller of the two? _fibula_____

10. Which of the bones of the distal leg is located laterally? _FIBULA_____

11. Which bone of the distal leg is located more posteriorly? _FIBULA_____

12. What is the term describing the most distal portion of the fibula? (a) _LATERAL MALLEOLUS_,

    (b) the most distal tibia? _MEDIAL MALLEOLUS_____

13. What are the names of the small round bones located near the metatarsophalangeal joints? _____

    _sesamoid_____

14. The transverse arch of the foot is primarily formed by which four bones? A. _1ST CUNEIFORM_

    B. _2ND CUNEIFORM_   C. _3RD CUNEIFORM_   D. _CUBOID_

15. Write the second term used to describe the following surfaces and projections of the foot:

    A. Dorsal surface _anterior_____

    B. Posterior surface _plantar_____

    C. PA projection _plantodorsal_____

    D. Dorsoplantar projection _AP_____

16. A tri-malleolar fracture involves which bones? _Tibia fibula calcaneus_

MEDIAL LATERAL + POSTERIOR MALLEOLI OF TIBIA & FIBULA

17. The inferior portions of the tibia and fibula form a deep socket called the _ANKLE MORTISE_.

18. Write the correct classifications, mobility and movement type for the following joints:

	Structural Classification	Mobility Type	Movement Type
A. Ankle	(a) _SYNOVIAL_	(b) _DIARTHRODIAL_	(c) _HINGE_
B. Interphalangeal	(a) _SYNOVIAL_	(b) _DIARTHRODIAL_	(c) _HINGE_
C. Intertarsal	(a) _SYNOVIAL_	(b) _DIARTHRODIAL_	(c) _GLIDING_
D. Tarsometatarsal joints	(a) _SYNOVIAL_	(b) _DIARTHRODIAL_ _freely moving_	(c) _GLIDING_

19. Fill in the following from the labeled drawings: (List both terms where indicated)

A. _calcaneus (os calcis)_

B. _talus (ASTRAGALUS)_

C. _navicular (scaphoid)_

D. _cuneiform 2nd_

E. _cuneiform 1st_

F. _1st metatarsal_

G. _MP joint 1st_

H. _proximal phalanx_

I. _middle PROXIMAL IP joint 2nd PIP_

J. _middle phalanx 5th_

K. _5th MP joint_

L. _head of 5th metatarsal_

M. _5th metatarsal (shaft)_

N. _base of 5th metatarsal_

O. _CUBOID_

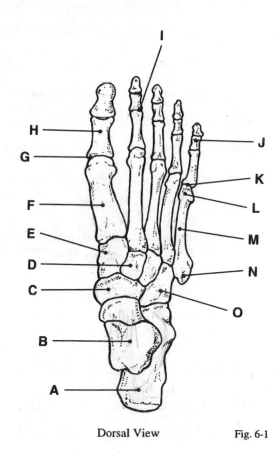

Dorsal View   Fig. 6-1

19. (*continued*)

P. _TALUS_   ASTRAGALUS

Q. _CALCANEUS_   OS CALCIS

R. _CUBOID_

S. _BASE OF 5th METATARSAL_

T. _1st MEDIAL CUNEIFORM_

U. _NAVICULAR_

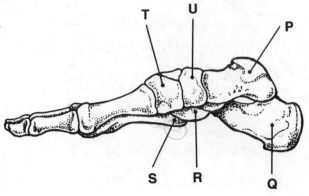

Medial View   Fig. 6-2

V. _TIBIA_

W. _MEDIAL MALLEOLUS_

X. _TALUS_   astragalus

Y. _LATERAL MALLEOLUS_

Z. _FIBULA_

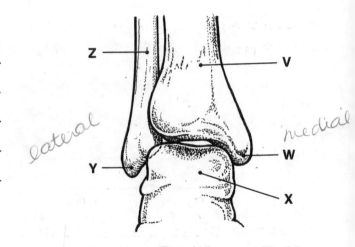

Frontal View   Fig. 6-3

20. Identify the labeled parts of the calcaneus and distal leg and foot from the following two drawings.

A. _SUSTENTACULUM TALI_

B. _TALOCALCANEAL JOINT_ (subtalar)

C. _TUBEROSITY_

D. _LATERAL PROCESS_

E. _PERONEAL TROCHLEA_

F. _LATERAL MALLEOLUS OF FIBULA_

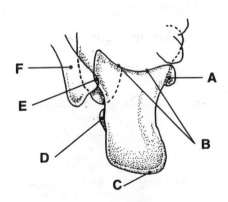

Plantodorsal Projection
or View   Fig. 6-4

20. *(continued)*

G. LATERAL MALLEOLUS OF FIBULA

H. TIBIOTALAR JOINT

I. CALCANEUS ✓

J. TUBEROSITY ─

K. TALOCALCANEAL JOINT

L. CALCANEOCUBOID JOINT

M. TALONAVICULAR JOINT ✓

N. TALUS ✓

O. TARSAL SINUS ✓

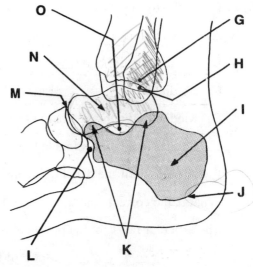

Lateral Aspect or View   Fig. 6-5

21. Identify the bones with which each of the following tarsals articulate:

A. Calcaneus (a) CUBOID   (b) TALUS

B. Talus   (a) TIBIA   (b) FIBULA

          (c) CALCANEUS   (d) NAVICULAR

C. Navicular (a) TALUS   (b) three CUNEIFORMS

D. 1st, medial cuneiform (a) NAVICULAR   (b) 1ST METATARSAL

               (c) 2ND METATARSAL (d) 2ND CUNEIFORM

E. 2nd, intermediate cuneiform (a) NAVICULAR   (b) 2ND METATARSAL

               (c) 1ST 2ND CUNEIFORM (d) 3RD CUNEIFORM

F. Cuboid (a) CALCANEUS   (b) 3RD LATERAL CUNEIFORM

        (c) 4th METATARSAL   (d) 5th METATARSAL

Review Exercise B   Anatomy of Leg, Knee, Patella, and Femur

Textbook: pp 176-182
Audio-visuals: Unit 8, slides 1-20

1. Fill in the following for the two bones of the lower leg (tibia or fibula):

   A. Larger, weight-bearing bone ___tibia___

   B. Smaller, "calf" bone ___fibula___

   C. Medial bone ___tibia___

   D. Medial malleolus refers to the distal ___tibia___.

   E. Lateral malleolus refers to the distal ___fibula___. ✓

   F. A fracture of the distal tibia, often also indicates a possible fracture to the ___PROX. FIBULA___.

2. What is the correct anatomical term for "tibial spine?" ___INTERCONDYLOID EMINENCE___

3. The articular facet for the proximal tibiofibular articulation is located on the (a) ___INFERIOR___ ___POSTERIOR___ aspect of the (b) ___LATERAL___ condyle of the (c) ___TIBIA___.

4. What is the condition or disease called when the tibial tuberosity breaks away from the tibia? ___Osgood-Schlatter___

5. List all the joints described in this chapter (foot, ankle, leg, knee and <u>distal</u> femur) for the following movement type and classifications:

   A. Ball and socket joint(s) ___-NONE-___

   B. Hinge joint(s) ___IP, KNEE, ANKLE___

   C. Gliding type(s) ___PROX TIB-FIB, INTERTARSAL, TARSOMETATARSAL___

   D. Diarthrodial joint(s) ___ALL OF LOWER LIMB EXCEPT DISTAL TIB-FIB___

   E. Amphiarthrodial joint(s) ___DISTAL TIB-FIB___

   F. Synovial joint(s) ___ALL___

6. The largest, strongest bone in the human body is the ___femur___.

7. The deep depression between the condyles of the distal femur is called the (a) ___INTERCONDYLOID FOSSA___ and is located on the (b) ___POSTERIOR DISTAL FEMUR___.

8. The patella is classified as what type of bone? ___sesamoid___

9. Describe how you would locate the knee joint for positioning for an AP projection using the patella as a reference. ___½" below the patella (1 cm)___

10. The posterior aspect of the knee is referred to as the ___popliteal___ region.

11. Stress views of the knee are taken primarily to check for damage to the ___tendons KNEE LIGAMENTS___

12. The structures acting as "shock absorbers" in the knee joint are called ~~bursae~~ <u>MENISCI</u>

13. Fill in the following from the labeled drawings.
(List two terms where indicated.)

A. <u>INTERCONDYLOID EMINENCE</u> (<u>TIBIAL SPINE</u>)

B. <u>MEDIAL CONDYLE OF TIBIA</u>

C. <u>ARTICULAR FACETS</u> (<u>TIBIAL PLATEAU</u>)

D. <u>TIBIAL TUBEROSITY</u>

E. <u>SHAFT OF TIBIA</u> (<u>DIAPHYSIS</u>)

F. <u>MEDIAL MALLEOLUS OF TIBIA</u>

G. <u>LATERAL MALLEOLUS OF FIBULA</u>

H. <u>BODY OR SHAFT OF FIBULA</u>

I. <u>HEAD OF FIBULA</u>

J. <u>STYLOID PROCESS OF FIBULA</u> (<u>APEX</u>)

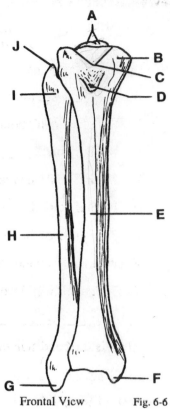

Frontal View   Fig. 6-6

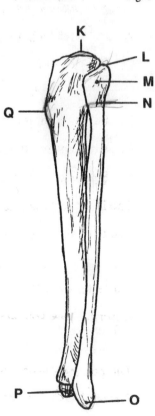

K. <u>INTERCONDYLOID EMINENCE</u> (<u>TIBIAL SPINE</u>)

L. <u>APEX OF FIBULA</u> (<u>STYLOID PROCESS</u>)

M. <u>HEAD OF FIBULA</u>

N. <u>NECK OF FIBULA</u>

O. <u>LATERAL MALLEOLUS OF FIBULA</u>

P. <u>MEDIAL MALLEOLUS OF TIBIA</u>

Q. <u>TIBIAL TUBEROSITY</u>

Lateral Aspect or View   Fig. 6-7

14. Identify the following parts from these drawings of the knee:

A. ~~FEMUR~~ ✓

B. ~~PATELLA~~

C. ~~MEDIAL CONDYLE~~ ✓

D. ~~TIBIAL PLATEAU (ARTICULAR FACETS)~~ ✓

E. ~~PROX. TIB-FIB JOINT~~ ✓

F. ~~FIBULA~~ ~~TIBIA~~

G. ~~NECK OF FIBULA~~ ✓

H. ~~HEAD OF FIBULA~~ ✓

I. ~~LATERAL CONDYLE OF TIBIA~~

J. ~~LATERAL CONDYLE OF FEMUR~~ ✓

K. ~~PATELLOFEMORAL JOINT~~ ✓

L. ~~INTERCONDYLOID EMINENCE (TIBIAL SPINE)~~ ✓

M. ~~TIBIA~~ ✓

N. ~~FIBULA~~ ✓

O. ~~HEAD OF FIBULA~~ ✓

P. ~~MEDIAL & LATERAL CONDYLES (SUPERIMPOSED)~~ ✓

Q. ~~FEMUR~~ ✓

Medial Oblique
Position or View   Fig. 6-8

Lateral Position
or View   Fig. 6-9

15. Identify the following four major ligaments which provide stability for the knee joint:

A. The two large ligaments on each side of the knee preventing abduction and adduction movements of the knee are:

~~FIBULAR~~ and ~~TIBIAL COLLATERAL LIGAMENTS~~

B. The two strong ligaments which lie within the capsule or knee joint preventing anterior or posterior displacement of the knee joint are:

~~ANTERIOR~~ and ~~POSTERIOR CRUCIATE LIGAMENTS~~

16. A blow to the lateral side of the knee such as a football injury would most likely rupture the ~~TIBIAL COLLATERAL~~ ligament.

17. A direct blow to the anterior knee would most likely rupture or damage the ~~POSTERIOR CRUCIATE~~ ligament.

Part II. RADIOGRAPHIC POSITIONING

Review Exercise C   Positioning of Toes, Foot, Calcaneus, and Ankle

Textbook: pp 183-200
Audio-visuals: Unit 7, slides 27-60

1. List the basic projections and the central ray location for the following:

	Basic Projections	Central Ray
A. Toe (5th digit)	(a) _AP, lateral, obl_	(b) _prox IP_
B. Foot	(a) _AP, obl, lat_	(b) _base of 3rd metatarsal_
C. Calcaneus	(a) _lat, axial_	(b) _base of 3rd metatarsal_
D. Ankle	(a) _AP, obl, lat (AP mortise)_	(b) _mid-ankle_

9 ✓
2+9×9 (LAT)
7×9
2+9×9 (LAT)

2. For oblique and lateral projections of the 3rd and 4th digits of the foot, the foot should be rotated **laterally or medially?** _laterally_

3. Indicate which rotation and how many degrees should be used on an oblique foot: (a) _45° medially_   *45°MEDIALLY*   *10°-15° med*

    oblique ankle: (b) _45° medially_ 5°-10°   *45°MEDIALLY*

    oblique mortise position for ankle: (c) _15°-20° medially_   *91*

4. The plantodorsal projection of the calcaneus requires a (a) _40_ degree angle from the

    (b) _plantar surface_ of the foot.   *cephalic*

5. The plantodorsal projection of the calcaneus requires an **increase** or **decrease** (a) _increase_

    of about (b) _4-6_ kVp from an AP foot or ankle?

6. What are the basic projections for an ankle in a cast? _AP & lateral_

    all parts → AP - lateral - 2 views 90° apart

7. Indicate how much you would increase exposure factors from a routine ankle to a post-reduction ankle

    in a fiberglass cast (a) _3-4 kVp_, in a dry plaster cast (b) _5-7 kVp_, or in a large or

    wet plaster cast (c) _8-10 kVp or 2× mAs_.

8. True or False: (Explain why) The malleoli of the ankle should be used for positioning for an AP

    ankle by insuring that they are the same distance from the film? _false_

    lateral will be more posterior

9. A grid should be used for all body parts measuring over _10- 13_ cm.

10. Describe positioning of the ankle to best demonstrate an "opened" view of the mortise joint:

ROTATE LEG + FOOT INWARD 15-20° .... OBLIQUE

11. Which lateral projection is recommended for a routine lateral foot (mediolateral or lateromedial)?

A. *mediolateral*

B. Why? *more comfortable for patient*

12. Describe the CR angle for routine projections of the following:

A. AP toe ___*−none−*___ ** *10°-15° cephalic*

B. AP foot ___*10°−15° cephalic*___

C. AP ankle stress projections ___*90° to none*___

D. Lateral foot ___*none*___

E. Plantodorsal (axial) projection of calcaneus ___*40° cephalic*___

F. Oblique foot ___*−none−*___

G. AP ankle mortise position ___*−none−*___

Review Exercise D   Positioning of Leg, Knee, Patella, and Femur   Textbook: pp 202-216
Audio-visuals: Unit 8, slides 21-59

1. List the basic projections and the size and type of film holder

		Basic Projections		Number, Size & Type of Film Holder(s) (screen or grids)
A.	Leg	(a) *AP, late*	(b) *14×17 or 2 7×17 Screens* *7×17 10×12 for an* *CR mid shaft*
B.	Knee - Routine	(a) *PA (trauma) 9×9* *AP, obl, lat, axial* *(non-trauma) (tunnel)*	(b) *10×12 in bucky* *CR to bend of leg*
C.	Patella	(a) *PA, lat, axial*	(b) *9×9*
D.	Distal half of femur	(a) *AP, lat*	(b) *14×17 or ≠7×17*
E.	Intercondyloid fossa *tunnel*	(a) *PA, axial*	(b) *8×10*

2. List the structures and/or joints best demonstrated on the following:

   A. Medial oblique knee (AP) _prox tib-fib ° lateral condyles_
      without superimposition

   B. Tangential (axial) projection for patella _patellofemoral joint space_
      + intercondyloid sulcus

   C. PA axial (tunnel view) _intercondyloid fossa, intercondyloid_
      eminence ° articular facets of tibia

   D. Lateral patella _patella in profile and_
      patellofemoral joint

3. List four names describing different tangential (axial) projections of the patella and patellofemoral joint

   A. _merchant_   B. _erect position_   C. _Hughston_
   D. _Settegast_

4. Why is it especially important to include both knee and ankle joints on an initial trauma AP and lateral leg?
   trauma to distal leg → proximal fibula fracture

5. Why should routine knee projections always be taken before positioning the patient for the Settegast position? _to make sure the patella isn't fractured_

6. Which rotation and how many degrees should be used for a routine AP oblique projection of knee?
   45° internal rotation

7. When radiographing the femur, why is it especially important to use gonad shields in addition to good close collimation? _close proximity of gonadal area_

8. Answer the following for a lateral knee projection:

   A. Which way should the knee be rotated (internally or externally for lateromedial or mediolateral)?
      external- mediolateral

   B. Approximately how much should the knee be flexed? _15°-20°_

   C. List two reasons why the knee should not be flexed to 45 or even 90 degrees for this lateral
      projection? (a) _tighten muscles -draw patella in_ and
      (b) _separation of patellar fractures_

   D. How much and which direction should the CR be angled? _5°-10° cephalic_

   E. A short heavy-set patient would require (a) _10_ degree CR angle and a tall thin patient
      would require (b) _5_ degrees.

Review Exercise E   Laboratory Activity   Textbook: pp. 187-216

This part of the learning activity exercises needs to be carried out in an x-ray laboratory or a general diagnostic room in a radiology department. Part B can be carried out in a classroom or any room where illuminators are available.

A. Positioning Exercise

For this section you need another person to act as your patient. Practice the following until you can do each of them accurately and without hesitation. It is important to achieve both accuracy and speed in radiographic positioning. Place a check by each when you have achieved this.

Include the following details as you simulate the basic projections for each exam listed below:

- patient shielding as needed
- correct size and type of film holder
- correct location of central ray and correct centering of part to film
- correct placement of markers
- accurate collimation
- proper use of immobilizing devices when needed
- approximate correct exposure factors
- correct instructions to your patient as you simulate the exposure

__   1. First digit of foot

__   2. Third digit of foot

__   3. Foot

__   4. Calcaneus

__   5. Ankle

__   6. Ankle in cast

__   7. Leg

__   8. Knee

__   9. Patella

__   10. Intercondyloid fossa

__   11. Mid and distal femur

Optional: Using either a sectional or fully articulated phantom, produce a diagnostic radiograph for each basic projection for the following:

__   1. Foot

__   2. Calcaneus

__   3. Ankle

__   4. Leg

__   5. Knee

__   6. Mid and distal femur

B. Review of Anatomy

Use those radiographs provided by your instructor.

___ 1.　Examine radiographs for each of the examinations listed in Part A, and identify all anatomical parts of the lower limb. Include all joints, phalanges, metatarsals, tarsals, and the bones involved in the ankle and knee joints.

C. Film Critique and Evaluation

Your instructor will provide various radiographs of the lower limb for these exercises. Some will be optimal quality radiographs meeting all or most of the evaluation criteria described for each projection in the textbook and/or audio-visuals. Others will be less than optimal quality and several will be unacceptable, requiring a repeat exam. You should evaluate each radiograph as specified below.

Place a check by each of the following when it is completed.

___ 1.　Critique each radiograph based on evaluation criteria provided for each projection in the textbook and/or audio-visuals. The following criteria guidelines can be used and checked as each radiograph is evaluated. (Additional checks can be placed to the left for each criteria guideline if more than six radiographs are evaluated.)

　　　Radiographs　　　　　　　　Criteria Guidelines
　1　2　3　4　5　6

__ __ __ __ __ __　a. Correct film size and correct orientation of part to film?

__ __ __ __ __ __　b. Correct alignment and/or centering of part to film or portion of film being used?

__ __ __ __ __ __　c. Correct collimation and CR location?

__ __ __ __ __ __　d. Pertinent anatomy well visualized?

__ __ __ __ __ __　e. Motion?

__ __ __ __ __ __　f. Optimum exposure; density and/or contrast?

__ __ __ __ __ __　g. Patient ID information and markers?

___ 2.　Based on acceptable variances to criteria factors, determine which of these radiographs are acceptable and which are unacceptable and should have been repeated.

Important:　　It is important that you have successfully carried out all of the exercises described above before taking the self-test and before going to your instructor for the chapter evaluation exam. If you neglect these exercises, you will not be able to meet all the objectives for this chapter and may not receive a passing grade for this course.

Answers to Review Exercise A

1. A. 14
   B. 5
   C. 7
   D. 26

2. A. Distal and proximal phalanx
   B. Distal, middle and proximal phalanx

3. A. Interphalangeal joint or IP joint
   B. Distal and proximal interphalangeal joints, or DIP & PIP joints
   C. Talocalcaneal (subtalar) joint
   D. Ankle

4. A. Five metatarsals
   B. Medially

5. A. Base
   B. Shaft
   C. Head

6. A. Three
   B. Tarsal sinus or sinus tarsi

7. A. Calcaneus or os calcis
   B. Talus or astragalus
   C. Calcaneus or os calcis
   D. Talus or astragalus
   E. Navicular or scaphoid
   F. 1. First, medial (internal) cuneiform
      2. Second intermediate (middle) cuneiform
      3. Third lateral (external) cuneiform
      4. Cuboid
      5. Cuboid

8. A. Talus
   B. Tibia
   C. Fibula

9. Fibula

10. Fibula

11. Fibula

12. (a) lateral malleolus (b) medial malleolus

13. Sesamoid bones

14. A. 1st (internal) cuneiform
    B. 2nd (middle) cuneiform
    C. 3rd (external) cuneiform
    D. cuboid

15. A. Anterior
    B. Plantar
    C. Plantodorsal
    D. AP

16. Medial, lateral and posterior malleoli, of tibia and fibula

17. ankle mortise

18. A. (a) synovial (b) diarthrodial (c) hinge
    B. (a) synovial (b) diarthrodial (c) hinge
    C. (a) synovial (b) diarthrodial (c) gliding
    D. (a) synovial (b) diarthrodial (c) gliding

19. A. Calcaneus (os calcis)
    B. Talus (astragalus)
    C. Navicular (scaphoid)
    D. Second intermediate (middle) cuneiform
    E. First medial (internal) cuneiform
    F. First metatarsal
    G. First MP or metatarsophalangeal joint
    H. Proximal phalanx, first digit of right foot
    I. Proximal interphalangeal (PIP) joint, 2nd digit of right foot
    J. Middle phalanx, 5th digit of right foot
    K. 5th metatarsophalangeal joint, right foot
    L. Head of 5th metatarsal
    M. Shaft or diaphysis of 5th metatarsal
    N. Base of 5th metatarsal (tuberosity)
    O. Cuboid
    P. Talus or astragalus
    Q. Calcaneus or os calcis
    R. Cuboid
    S. Base of 5th metatarsal (tuberosity)
    T. First medial (internal)
    U. Navicular or scaphoid
    V. Tibia
    W. Medial malleolus
    X. Talus
    Y. Lateral malleolus
    Z. Fibula

Answers to Review Exercise A continued

20. A. Sustentaculum tali
     B. Talocalcaneal joint
     C. Tuberosity
     D. Lateral process
     E. Peroneal trochlea (trochlear process)
     F. Lateral malleolus of fibula

     G. Lateral malleolus of fibula
     H. Tibiotalar joint
     I. Calcaneus
     J. Tuberosity
     K. Talocalcaneal (subtalar) joint
     L. Calcaneocuboid joint
     M. Talonavicular joint
     N. Talus
     O. Tarsal sinus

21. A. (a) cuboid   (b) talus
     B. (a) tibia   (b) fibula   (c) calcaneus
         (d) navicular
     C. (a) talus (b) cuneiforms
     D. (a) navicular (b) 1st metatarsal
         (c) 2nd metatarsal
         (d) 2nd, intermediate cuneiform
     E. (a) navicular (b) 2nd metatarsal
         (c) 2nd, medial cuneiform
         (d) 3rd, lateral cuneiform
     F. (a) calcaneus
         (b) 3rd, lateral cuneiform
         (c) 4th metatarsal (d) 5th metatarsal

If you missed more than 20 blanks, you should review this section again in the textbook and/or audio-visuals before continuing.

Answers to Review Exercise B

1. A. Tibia
    B. Fibula
    C. Tibia
    D. Tibia
    E. Fibula
    F. Proximal fibula

2. Intercondyloid eminence

3. (a) inferior posterior (b) lateral
    (c) tibia

4. Osgood-Schlatter disease

5. A. None (hip joint would be ball and
       socket joint involving lower limb)
    B. Knee, ankle, and interphalangeal
       joints
    C. Proximal tibiofibular articulation,
       intertarsal and tarsometatarsal joints
    D. All joints of lower limb except distal
       tibiofibular joint
    E. Distal tibiofibular articulation
    F. All joints of lower limb

6. Femur

7. (a) intercondyloid fossa or notch,
    (b) posterior aspect of the distal femur

8. Sesamoid

9. The knee joint is one-half inch or one
    centimeter below apex of patella.

10. Popliteal region

11. Knee ligaments

12. Menisci

13. A. Intercondyloid eminence (tibial spine)
    B. Medial condyle of tibia
    C. Articular facets (tibial plateau)
    D. Tibial tuberosity
    E. Shaft (diaphysis) of tibia
    F. Medial malleolus of tibia
    G. Lateral malleolus of fibula
    H. Body or shaft of fibula
    I. Head of fibula
    J. Styloid process (apex) of fibula

13. (*continued*)

    K. Intercondyloid eminence (tibial spine)
    L. Apex of fibula (styloid process)
    M. Head of fibula
    N. Neck of fibula
    O. Lateral malleolus of fibula
    P. Medial malleolus of tibia
    Q. Tibial tuberosity

14. A. Femur
    B. Patella
    C. Medial condyle
    D. Tibial plateau (articular facets)
    E. Proximal tibiofibular joint
    F. Fibula
    G. Neck of fibula
    H. Head of fibula
    I. Lateral condyle of tibia
    J. Lateral condyle of femur

    K. Patellofemoral joint
    L. Intercondyloid eminence
    M. Tibia
    N. Fibula
    O. Head of fibula
    P. Superimposed medial and lateral
       condyles
    Q. Femur

15. A. Fibular and tibial collateral ligaments
    B. Anterior and posterior cruciate
       ligaments

16. Tibial collateral ligament

17. Posterior cruciate ligament

If you missed more than 15 blanks, you should review
this section again in the textbook and/or audio-visuals
before continuing.

Answers to Review Exercise C

1. A. (a) AP, obli. and lat.
    B. (a) AP, obli. and lat.
    C. (a) Plantodorsal and lat.
    D. (a) AP, AP mortise, obli. and lat.

    (b) PIP or proximal interphalangeal joint
    (b) base of 3rd metatarsal
    (b) base of 3rd metatarsal and mid calcaneus
    (b) mid ankle joint

2. Laterally

3. (a) 45° medially (b) 45° medially
    (c) 15-20° medially

4. (a) 40 (b) plantar surface or long axis

5. (a) increase (b) 4-6

6. AP and lateral, or two projections 90 degrees from each other

7. (a) 3-4 kVp
    (b) 5-7 kVp
    (c) 8-10 kVp

8. False (The lateral malleolus will be 15° more posterior)

9. 10

10. Rotate the leg and foot internally about 15-20° until the intermalleolar line is parallel to the film.

11. A. Mediolateral
    B. It is less painful for patient

12. A. 10-15° cephalad (toward calcaneus)
    B. 10° cephalad (toward calcaneus)
    C. 90° to film (none)
    D. 90° to film (none)
    E. 40° cephalad
    F. 90° to film (none)
    G. 90° to film (none)

If you missed more than 6 blanks, you should review this section again in the textbook and/or audio-visuals before continuing.

Answers to Review Exercise D

1.   A.   (a) AP and lat.   (b) 1 - 14 x 17 or 2 - 7 x 17 screens
        B.   (a) AP, obli. (with 45 degree internal rotation) and lat.
             (b) 3 - 8 x 10 grids (or screens if less than 10 cm)
        C.   (a) PA, lat. and tangential (axial)   (b) grids for PA and lat.; if over 10 cm, screen for tangential.
        D.   (a) AP and lat.   (b) 2 - 14 x 17 or 2 -7 x 17
        E.   (a) PA and axial   (b) 2 - 8 x 10 grids (screen if less than 10 cm)

2.   A.   Proximal tibiofibular joint and lateral condyles of femur and tibia without superimposition.
        B.   Patellofemoral joint space and intercondyloid sulcus (trochlear groove)
        C.   Intercondyloid fossa, intercondyloid eminence and articular facets of tibia
        D.   Patella in profile and patellofemoral joint

3.   A.   Merchant method   B.   Erect position method   C.   Hughston method
        D.   Settegast method

4.   Fracture or trauma to distal leg frequently is associated with a second fracture of proximal fibula (and for legal purposes).

5.   To rule out transverse fracture of patella.

6.   Forty-five degrees internal rotation.

7.   Because of proximity to reproductive organs.

8.   A.   Externally for mediolateral projection
        B.   15-20 degrees
        C.   (a) Additional flexion will tighten muscles and draw patella into intercondylar sulcus thus obscuring soft tissue information.
             (b) May cause separation of patellar fractures if present.
        D.   5-10 degrees cephalad
        E.   (a) 10
             (b) 5

If you missed more than 5 blanks, you should review this section again in the textbook and/or audio-visuals before continuing.

Self-Test

My score = _____ %

Directions: Take this self-test only after completing all the review exercises and laboratory activities in this chapter. Complete directions including grading requirements are described in the front pages of this workbook and in the self-test of Chapter 1.

Test

There are 100 blanks. Each correct blank is worth 1 point. (Spelling is important so correct any misspellings as you grade your test.)

1. The digits of the foot are made up of fourteen separate bones called the __phalanges__.

2. How many tarsals are present in the foot? __7__

3. Write in the correct names for the bones making up the following: (starting with the proximal bone)

   A. 1st digit (a) __prox phalanx,__ and (b) __distal phalanx__

   B. 4th digit (a) __prox phalanx__, (b) __middle phalanx__

   and (c) __distal phalanx__.

4. Name the three parts of each metatarsal.

   A. __base__ _PROXIMAL_

   B. __shaft (DIAPHYSIS)__

   C. __head__

5. Which tarsal is directly involved in the ankle joint? __talus__ __astragus__ _ASTRAGALUS_

6. What is the correct name for each of the following joints? (Use both initials and names where applicable.)

   A. Between 1st metatarsal and proximal phalanx __metatarsal phalangeal MTP__ _METATARSOPHALANGEAL_

   B. Between proximal and middle phalanx, 2nd digit __prox IP__

   C. Between talus and calcaneus __talocalcaneal (SUBTALAR)__

   D. Between tarsals and metatarsal __tarsalmetatarsal__ _TARSOMETATARSAL_

7. The name of the small bones usually present on the posterior aspect of the 1st metatarsophalangeal joint?
   __sesamoid__

8. Write in the correct names of the following tarsals. (Include both names where indicated.)

    A.   Articulate with proximal end of 4th and 5th metatarsals _____ cuboidal _____

    B.   Articulate with tibia and fibula _____ talus _____ (astragalus)

    C.   Located between talus and cuneiforms _____ navicular _____ (scaphoid)

    D.   Largest tarsal _____ os calcis _____ (calcaneus)

    E.   Articulates with proximal end of 2nd metatarsal _____ 2nd cuneiform _____

9. The ankle joint is classified as a (a) _____ synovial _____ joint, with a (b) _____ diarthrodal _____

    mobility type , and a (c) _____ hinge _____ movement type.

10. Identify the labeled parts of this lateral ankle drawing:

    A. _____ tibia _____

    B. _____ ANTERIOR TUBERCLE OF TIBIA _____

    C. _____ TALOCALCANEAL JOINT _____ subtalar

    D. _____ navicular _____

    E. _____ CUBOID _____

    F. _____ BASE OF 5th METATARSAL _____

    G. _____ TARSAL SINUS _____

    H. _____ os calcis _____ CALCANEUS

    I. _____ talus _____ ASTRAGALUS

    J. _____ LATERAL MALLEOLUS _____ (fibula)

    K. _____ fibula _____

Lateral View   Fig. 6-10

11. List the correct central ray location for the following:

    A.   AP ankle _____ mid ankle joint _____

    B.   Lateral ankle _____ ankle joint _____ LATERAL MALLEOLUS

    C.   AP foot _____ base 3rd metatarsal _____

    D.   Plantodorsal of calcaneus _____ base of 3rd metatarsal _____

    E.   Lateral calcaneus _____ heel _____ MID CALCANEUS

    F.   2nd digit, right foot _____ prox IP joint _____

12. Matching: (choices on the right may be used more than once)

    _6_   A. Dorsum ✓   1. plantodorsal

    _5_   B. Plantar ✓   2. dorsoplantar

    _2_   C. AP ✓   3. calcaneus

    _1_   D. PA ✓   4. talus

    _4_   E. 2nd largest tarsal   5. posterior surface

   _~~10~~_   F. Dorsum (pedis)   6. anterior surface

    _3_   G. Heel bone ✓   7. tibia

    _3_   H. Os calcis ✓   8. fibula

    _4_   I. Astragalus   9. navicular

    _8_   J. Lateral malleolus _fibula_   10. cuboid

    _7_   K. Medial malleolus _tibia_   11. pisiform

7   ~~_8_~~   L. "Posterior" malleolus _tibia_ 12. amphiarthrodial

    _9_   M. Scaphoid   13. pivot joint

    _8_   N. Smaller bone of lower leg   ⟨14. hinge joint⟩

   _15_   O. Intertarsal joint   15. gliding joint

   _15_   P. Tarsometatarsal joint   16. saddle joint

-12 ~~_15_~~   Q. Distal tibiofibular joint _amphi_ ⟨17. hinge joint⟩

-16 ~~_14_~~   R. Patellofemoral joint _saddle_

17 ~~_15_~~   S. Tibiofemoral joint

17 ~~_14_~~ ok   T. Ankle joint

17 ~~_14_~~ ok   U. Interphalangeal joint

metatarsophalangeal – condyloid

13. List the degrees and the direction of angle for the following projections:

    A. AP foot _10 ~~15~~_ degrees, _cephalic_ angle

    B. Plantodorsal of calcaneus _40_ degrees, _cephalic_ angle

14. A sports injury of a blow to the lateral aspect of the knee is most likely to tear the _____ _tibial collateral_ ligament

15. The calcaneus articulates with the (a) _cuboid_ anteriorly and with the (b) _talus_ superiorly.

16. The navicular articulates with the _talus_ posteriorly.

True or False (Explain why):

17. To insure a true AP ankle, the intermalleolar line should be parallel to the film.
     false _lateral malleolus 15° more posterior_

18. A true lateral ankle or distal leg will position the distal fibula directly over the mid distal tibia. _____
     FALSE _FIBULA OVER POSTERIOR ½ to ⅔ OF TIBIA_

19. Gonadal shielding is needed on exams of the lower limb even if tight collimation is used.
     true ✓

20. A grid should always be used for exams of both the knee and the distal femur. _grid over 10cm_
     false – don't need a grid _screen for knees less th__ _10 c_

21. The lateromedial is the preferred projection for a lateral foot. _false – mediolateral_
     more comfortable for patient

22. A true AP projection of the ankle will "open up" the mortise joint of the ankle. _false –_
     oblique _15°–20°_

23. For the ankle mortise projection, the leg and foot should be rotated internally 15-20°.
     true _to open up ankle mortise – oblique_

Multiple choice (circle correct answers)

24. The navicular and the space between the 1st and 2nd metatarsals are best visualized on which oblique of the foot?

    a. 45° medial oblique
    b. 15° lateral oblique
    ~~c.~~ 15° medial oblique
    (d.) 30° lateral oblique

25. A true AP projection of the foot requires:

    a. CR 90° to film, no rotation of foot
    b. CR 10° cephalad, 5 to 10 degrees medial rotation of foot
    ✓ (c.) CR 10° cephalad, no rotation of foot
    d. CR 15° caudal, no rotation of root

26. To best separate the bases of the 3rd to 5th metatarsals on an oblique foot, the foot should be:

    (a.) rotated medially 45°
    b. rotated laterally 30°
    ~~c.~~ rotated laterally 45°
    d. rotated medially 30°

27. To best demonstrate the sesamoids and the head of the first metatarsal:

    a. CR 45° cephalad with plantar surface of foot 15-20° from vertical
    (b.) CR 90° to film with plantar surface of foot 15-20° from vertical
    c. CR perpendicular to long axis of the first metatarsal
    d. CR 25° cephalad with plantar surface of foot 90° to film

28. The popliteal region refers to _back of the knee_

29. What is the name of the concave, articular surface of the proximal tibia? _ARTICULAR FACETS_ _TIBIAL PLATEAU_

30. What process or part of the tibia is important in diagnosing Osgood-Schlatter disease?
tibial spine _/TIBIAL TUBEROSITY_

31. The name of the two cartilaginous pads located on the tibial plateau which act as shock absorbers at the knee joint are called the (a) _MEDIAL MENISCUS_ and (b) _LATERAL MENISCUS_ .

32. Should the central ray be angled on an AP knee projection? If so, how many degrees and which direction?
NO- WE DON'T ANGLE AP KNEE _**5° CEPHALIC_

33. A. Where should the central ray be directed on an AP knee projection? _3/4" BELOW APEX_
(BOTTOM) OF PATELLA

    B. On a lateral knee projection? _3/4" BELOW FEMORAL EPICONDYLE_

34. Determination of direction of rotation on an oblique knee:

    A. An AP medial (internal) oblique knee refers to internal rotation of the **anterior** or **posterior** aspect of the knee? _ANTERIOR_

    B. A PA medial (internal) oblique knee refers to internal rotation of the **anterior** or **posterior** aspect of the knee? _ANTERIOR_

35. Describe the two obliques of the knee and proximal leg (tibia-fibula) which can be taken to best demonstrate the proximal tibiofibular articulation and fibular head.

    A. _45° internal rotation AP_

    B. _45° internal rotation PA_

36. What are two terms commonly used for the special projection to visualize the intercondyloid fossa?

    A. _tunnel_

    B. _axial_

37. How can you evaluate a lateral knee radiograph for a true lateral? _____
CONDYLES SUPERIMPOSED

38. A fracture to the distal tibia, also suggests a possible fracture to the _prox fibula_

Answers to Self-Test

1. Phalanges

2. Seven

3. A. (a) proximal phalanx
      (b) distal phalanx

   B. (a) proximal phalanx
      (b) middle phalanx
      (c) distal phalanx

4. A. Base
   B. Shaft (diaphysis)
   C. Head

5. Talus (astragalus)

6. A. MP or metatarsophalangeal
   B. PIP or proximal interphalangeal
   C. Talocalcaneal (subtalar) joint
   D. TM or tarsometatarsal

7. Sesamoid bones

8. A. Cuboid
   B. Talus (astragalus)
   C. Navicular (scaphoid)
   D. Calcaneus (os calcis)
   E. 2nd, intermediate cuneiform

9. (a) synovial (b) diarthrodial
   (c) hinge

10. A. Tibia
    B. Anterior tubercle of tibia
    C. Talocalcaneal joint
    D. Navicular
    E. Cuboid
    F. Base of 5th metatarsal
    G. Tarsus sinus
    H. Calcaneus
    I. Talus
    J. Lateral malleolus
    K. Fibula

11. A. Mid ankle joint
    B. Lateral malleolus
    C. Base of 3rd metatarsal
    D. Base of 3rd metatarsal
    E. Mid calcaneus
    F. PIP or proximal interphalangeal joint

12. A. 6   K. 7
    B. 5   L. 7
    C. 2   M. 9
    D. 1   N. 8
    E. 4   O. 15
    F. 7   P. 15
    G. 3   Q. 12
    H. 3   R. 16
    I. 4   S. 17
    J. 8   T. 17
               U. 17

13. A. 10, cephalic (toward heel)
    B. 40, cephalic

14. Tibial collateral

15. (a) cuboid (b) talus

16. Talus

17. False (The lateral malleolus will be about 15° more posterior)

18. False (Fibula will be over posterior 1/2 or 2/3 of tibia)

19. True (Gonadal shielding should be used to prevent exposure from secondary and scatter radiation)

20. False (A screen can be used on a knee of less than 10 cm.)

21. False (Mediolateral is preferred because it is less painful for patients)

22. False (A 15–20° internal rotation does this)

23. True (To "open up" the entire ankle mortise)

24. d

25. c

26. a

27. b

28. The posterior knee region

29. Tibial plateau

Answers to Self-Test continued

30. Tibial tuberosity

31. (a) medial meniscus, (b) lateral meniscus

32. Yes, 5 degrees cephalic or as needed to be perpendicular to the long axis of the tibia.

33. A.   3/4" (1cm) below apex of patella
    B.   3/4 to 1 inch below medial epicondyle

34. A.   Anterior
    B.   Anterior

35. A.   45° internal (medial) rotation PA
    B.   45° internal (medial) rotation AP

36. A.   Tunnel view
    B.   Axial projection

37. Posterior borders of the femoral medial and lateral condyles will be directly superimposed.

38. Proximal fibula

Chapter 7
Proximal Femur and Pelvis

Rationale

Positioning for hip examinations is more difficult than for most other parts of the lower limb because it is impossible to palpate the hip joint directly. It is also difficult to visualize the relative positions of anatomical structures of the hip. Thus it becomes very important that you learn the anatomy of the hip well. It is especially important that you learn the location of these structures and be able to relate them to other structures and landmarks which you can locate by direct palpation.

The sacroiliac joints of the pelvis are unique in shape and position and you must learn this anatomy well enough on drawings and radiographs so you will know what position the pelvis must be in to "open-up" and visualize these joints on radiographs.

Specific positioning exercises are described in your workbook which will guide you in positioning for each exam as described in this chapter. The film critique exercises will help you learn to critique and judge radiographs to determine how they can be improved. You will also learn how to evaluate as to whether they are of acceptable diagnostic quality or if they need to be repeated and improved.

Successful completion of all exercises in this chapter should provide you with enough knowledge and skill to perform actual radiographic examinations on patients under the supervision of a technologist.

Chapter Objectives

After you have completed **all** the activities of this unit, you will be able, with at least 80% accuracy, to: (applicable to a written and/or oral examination and demonstration)

__1.   Identify, both on drawings and radiographs, all anatomy of the hips and pelvis as described in the textbook and/or audio-visuals.

__2.   Identify and locate on a patient the five positioning landmarks of the pelvis.

__3.   List the two divisions or cavities of the pelvis and describe the structural and functional differences of these two divisions.

__4.   List and describe three differences between the structure of the male and female pelvis.

__5.   Identify the correct classification and movement type for the joints of the pelvis.

__6.   Identify the structure of the proximal femur used as a key indicator on the radiograph to determine sufficient internal rotation of the legs to achieve a true AP hip projection.

__7.   Determine the specific rotation position of the leg based on the appearance of the proximal femur.

___ 8. List the basic projections, type and size of film holder, central ray location and anatomy best demonstrated for radiographic examinations of the hips, pelvis and sacroiliac joints.

___ 9. Position on a model and/or phantom the basic projections for the hips, pelvis and sacroiliac joints.

Given several radiographs of the hips, pelvis and sacroiliac joints:

___ 10. Determine the sex of patients from radiographs of the pelvis.

___ 11. Determine if rotation is present on radiographs of the pelvis.

___ 12. Critique each radiograph based on evaluation criteria provided in the textbook and/or audio-visuals.

___ 13. Discriminate between acceptable and unacceptable radiographs, based on exposure factors, collimation and positioning errors.

___ 14. Given the necessary equipment and a simulated patient (articulated phantom), produce a diagnostic radiograph for the basic projections of the hips, pelvis and sacroiliac joints.

Prerequisite

The prerequisite knowledge requirement for this chapter is an understanding of radiographic terminology and the principles of exposure, radiation protection and positioning as described in Chapter 1. It is strongly suggested that a mandatory prerequisite for this chapter be the successful completion of Chapter 1.

Recommended Supplementary References

The following supplementary references, which are described in more detail in Chapter 1, are listed in a suggested order of importance and value to understanding this material.

1. *Merrill's ...*, Vol 1, pp 242-277

2. *Clark's ...*, pp 124-142

3. *Eisenberg ...*, pp 136-148

Learning Activity Exercises

The following review exercises should be completed only after careful study of the associated pages in the textbook and/or audio-visuals as indicated by each exercise.

After completing each of these individual exercises, check your answers with the answer sheets which follow before continuing to the next exercise.

Part I. RADIOGRAPHIC ANATOMY

Review Exercise A Anatomy of Hips and Pelvis   Textbook: pp 217-224
                                                          Audio-visuals: Unit 9, slides 1-35

1. The two bones making up the **pelvic girdle** are (a) _left os coxa   LEFT HIP BONE_
   and (b) _right os coxa RIGHT HIP BONE_

2. The four bones comprising the **pelvis** are (a) _left os coxa_,
   (b) _sacrum_, (c) _coccyx_, and (d) _right os coxa_.

3. The two additional terms sometimes used for "hip bone" are (a) _INNOMINATE BONE_
   or (b) _OS COXA_

4. The three divisions of the hip bone are (a) _ilium_, (b) _ischium_,
   and (c) _pubis_.

5. What is the name for the largest foramen in the human body? _obdurator foramen_

6. The fusion of the three parts of the hip bone takes place around what structure? _acetabulum_

7. The two primary parts of the ilium are (a) _body_ and (b) _ala (wing)_

8. The two important positioning landmarks of the ilium are (a) _crest_,
   and (b) _ASIS_

9. What is the prominent structure of the ischium located directly posterior and slightly inferior to the
   acetabulum? _ischial spine_

10. The two parts of the hip bone, each of which constitute 2/5 of the acetabulum are the (a) _____
    ilium 2/5 and (b) _ischium_ 2/5   1/5 pubis

11. What is the name of the most inferior structure of the pelvis? ~~pubis~~ ischial tuberosity

12. The crest of the ilium extends from the (a) _ASIS_ anterior superior iliac spine anteriorly,
    to the (b) _PSIS_ posterior superior iliac spine posteriorly.

13. What is the articulation between the two pubic bones? _symphysis pubis_

14. What is the function of the following two divisions of the pelvis?

A. Greater (false) pelvis ___support abdominal organs + fetus___ *bones iliac + sacrum*

B. Lesser (true) pelvis ___birth canal___ ___cavity___

15. The size of the triangular shaped outlet of the true *(lesser)* pelvis is determined by the distances between three

structures, which are (a) *right* ___ischial tuberosity___, (b) *left* ___ischial tuberosity___,

and (c) ___coccyx___.

16. The size of the birth canal is frequently evaluated by what type of procedure? ___ultrasound___

17. List three differences between the structure of the male and female pelvis and describe each.

	Difference		Description	
			Female	Male
A.	(a) general shape	(b) wider, deeper, more flared	(c) narrow, less flared	
B.	(a) angle of pubic arch	(b) more than 90° (obtuse)	(c) less than 90° (acute) ∧	
C.	(a) shape of inlet	(b) round	(c) oval or heart-shaped	

18. Identify the classifications and movement type (if any) of the articulations of the pelvis.

Articulation	(a) Structural Classification	(b) Mobility Classification	(c) Movement Type (if applicable)
A. Sacroiliac joints	(a) synovial	(b) amphiarthrodial	(c) none
B. Symphysis pubis	(a) ~~synovial~~ cartilagenous	(b) amphiarthrodial	(c) none
C. Hip joints	(a) synovial	(b) diarthrodial	(c) ball + socket

19. The lesser trochanter is located on which aspect of the femur? ___medial, posterior___

20. Describe how to locate the **neck** of the femur using landmarks on the pelvis. ___straight line between ASIS + symphysis — 2.5" below midpoint (perpendicular)___

21. How would the **head** of the femur be located using the above landmarks of the pelvis? ___1.5"___
___below midpoint of line___

22. How should the leg and foot be positioned to achieve a true AP projection of the proximal femur? ___
___internal rotation 15°-20°___

23. What structure of the hip can be used as a key indicator on the radiograph to determine sufficient internal rotation of legs to achieve a true AP of the hip? _lesser trochanter_

24. How can the above indicator be used? _true AP hip will not show lesser trochanter_

25. Fill in the following from the labeled drawing:

A. _sacrum_
B. _sacroiliac joint_
C. _Crest of ilium_
D. _ASIS_
E. _acetabulum_
F. _Obdurato foramen_
G. _superior ramis of pubis_
H. _symphysis pubis_
I. _Ischium (superior ramis)_
J. _ischial spine_
K. _coccyx_

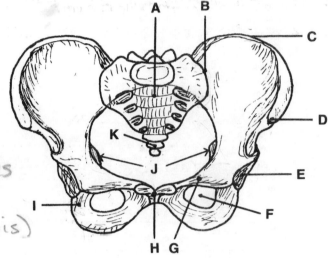

Frontal View of Pelvis   Fig. 7-1

L. _ASIS_
M. _ant. inf. iliac spine (AIIS)_
N. _ischial tuberosity_
O. _superior ramis of ischium_
P. _lesser sciatic notch_
Q. _ischial spine_
R. _greater sciatic notch_
S. _PIIS_
T. _PSIS_

Posterior   Anterior

Lateral View of   Fig. 7-2
Pelvic (Hip) Bone

25. *(continued)*

U. head
V. fovea capitis
W. neck
X. lesser trochanter
Y. intertrochanteric crest
Z. greater trochanter

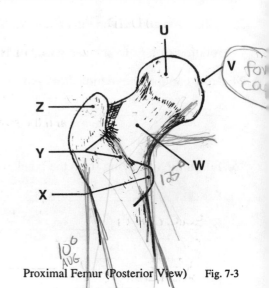

Proximal Femur (Posterior View)   Fig. 7-3

Anterior

a. femoral head
b. femoral neck
c. ischial tuberosity
d. acetabulum

Posterior

Axiolateral Hip   Fig. 7-4

10° avg
15° short female
5° tall male

26. The angle between the <u>neck</u> and the <u>shaft</u> of the femur on an average adult is about __125°__ degrees.

27. This angle would be **greater** or **lesser** on a short person with a wide pelvis? ~~greater~~ lesser
nearer vertical → greater angle

28. In the anatomical position the long axis of the femur is about (a) __15°__ degrees from vertical on a short
female, and (b) __5° 20°__ degrees on a tall slender male.   average adult 10°
(5°) pg. 218

29. In a true anatomical position on an average adult, the head of the femur is about __15°-20°__ degrees more
anterior than the body or shaft of the femur. (This is why the legs must be rotated internally for a true AP
hip and proximal femur.)

Part II   RADIOGRAPHIC POSITIONING

Review Exercise B   Positioning of Hips, Pelvis and Sacroiliac Joints

Textbook: pp 225-241
Audio-visuals: Unit 9, slides 36-64

1. List the basic projection(s) and the size, type and position of film holder(s) and the CR location for the following:

	Basic Projections (Include degrees of oblique if applicable)	ALL GRID Size, Type & Position of Film Holder	Central Ray Location (Include direction and degrees of angle if applicable)
A. Routine pelvis (no trauma)	(a) _AP pelvis_	(b) _14×17 crosswise_	(c) _center of pelvis_
B. Right hip (poss. fracture)	1 (a) _AP pelvis_ _shoot through_	1 (b) _14×17 crosswise_	(c) _left femoral neck_
	2 (a) _axiolateral_	2 (b) _8×10 lengthwise_	
C. Left hip (post reduction)	1 (a) _AP hip_	1 (b) _10×12 lengthwise_	(c) _left femoral neck_
	2 (a) _axiolateral_	2 (b) _8×10 lengthwise_	
D. Both hips (congenital dislocation)	1 (a) _AP pelvis_	1 (b) _14×17 crosswise_	(c) _femoral head_
	2 (a) _bilat frog leg_ _hips out_	2 (b) _14×17 crosswise_	
E. Sacroiliac joints	1 (a) _AP axial_	1 (b) _14×17 crosswise_	1 (c) _CR to center of pelvis 25° cephalic_
	2 (a) _25°-30° LPO + RPO_	2 (b) _a) 10×12 lengthwise_	2 (c) _CR to 1" medial upside ASIS_

2. What structures are best shown on an AP pelvis for both hips? _sacrum + coccyx,_ _pelvic girdle,   head, neck + greater trochanters of femur_

3. The two additional terms for an axiolateral hip projection are (a) _inferiosuperior_ and (b) _Danelius-Miller method_   _shoot through_

4. Where is the correct central ray location for an AP pelvis for both hips? _level of femoral heads, which is at upper margins of greater trochanters or 1½" above symphysis pubis_

5. Describe the most superior topographical landmark, and its relationship to the upper film margin, which should be used in positioning an AP pelvis.

   A. Topographical landmark _iliac crest_

   B. Relationship to upper film margin _top of film slightly above crest_

6. How could you evaluate for possible rotation on an AP pelvis radiograph? _obdurator foramen + ischial spines equal in size + shape + ala (wings of ilium)_

7. What is the best way to insure against rotation in positioning for an AP pelvis? _equal_ _distance from ASIS to table_

8. How should the legs and feet be positioned for a bilateral frog-leg hip projection? _flex both_ _knees + hips as far as possible_

9. Why should **both** hips be included on the AP projection if a possible fracture of only one hip is indicated? _comparison purposes_

10. Generally what would be the appearance of the leg and foot on a patient with a fracture of the left hip? _left leg + foot externally rotated_

11. What would be the appearance of the left hip on the radiograph of the above patient? _lesser_ _trochanter visible in profile on left femur_

12. True or False: (Indicate why.) For an AP pelvis and/or hip on a patient with a possible hip fracture, one should internally rotate both legs and feet about 10-20 degrees. _FALSE -_ _could displace femoral head + neck_

13. True or False: (Indicate why.) Gonad shields should always be used on both male and female patients of reproductive age or younger for a pelvis examination for possible hip fractures. _TRUE_ _close proximity_

14. Which sacroiliac joint is visualized on posterior obliques (the upside or the downside)? (a) _up side_   _LPO → right   RPO → left_   Which is visualized on anterior obliques? (b) _down side_ _LAO → left   RAO → right_

15. How many degrees and which oblique should be taken for:

   A. Left sacroiliac joint? (a) _25°- 30°_ degrees, (b) _RPO_ or (c) _LAO_

   B. Right sacroiliac joint? (a) _25°- 30°_ degrees, (b) _LPO_ or (c) _RAO_

16. Describe the patient position and CR location for an optional projection of the pelvis which could be taken to best demonstrate the left acetabulum and femoral head margin including the fovea capitis.

   A. Patient position _semi prone affected side down LAO_ _35°-40°_

   B. CR location _12° cephalic directed to acetabulum_

Review Exercise C Laboratory Activity   Textbook: pp 229-241

This part of the learning activity exercises needs to be carried out in an x-ray laboratory or a general diagnostic room in a radiology department. Part B can be carried out in a classroom or any room where illuminators are available.

A.   Positioning Exercise

For this section you need another person or an articulated phantom to act as your patient. Practice the following until you can do each of them accurately and without hesitation. It is important to achieve both accuracy and speed in radiographic positioning. Place a check by each when you have achieved this.

Include the following details as you simulate the basic projections for each exam listed below:

- correct size and type of film holder
- correct location of central ray and correct centering of part to film
- correct placement of markers
- accurate collimation
- proper use of immobilizing devices when needed
- approximate correct exposure factors
- correct instructions to your patient as you simulate the exposure
- use of gonadal shields when possible

___   1.   Pelvis (possible injury to general pelvis, not hips)

___   2.   Bi-lateral hips (8 year old patient for congenital hip problems)

___   3.   Left hip (possible fracture)

___   4.   Left hip (post reduction-hip nailing)

___   5.   Sacroiliac joints

Optional: Using either a sectional or fully articulated phantom, produce a diagnostic radiograph for each basic projection for the following:

___   1. Pelvis

___   2. Sacroiliac joints

B.   Review of Anatomy on Radiographs

Use those radiographs provided by your instructor. (These should include good radiographs of the pelvis, axiolateral hips, frog-leg hips and sacroiliac joints.)

___   1.   Examine radiographs of the pelvis and hips and identify all those anatomical parts described in the textbook and/or audio-visuals.

C. Film Critique and Evaluation

Your instructor will provide various radiographs of the pelvis, hips and sacroiliac joints for these exercises. Some will be optimum quality radiographs meeting all or most of the evaluation criteria described for each projection in the textbook and/or audio-visuals. Others will be less than optimum quality and several will be unacceptable, requiring a repeat exam. You should evaluate each radiograph as specified below.

Place a check by each of the following when it is completed.

___ 1. Critique each radiograph based on evaluation criteria provided for each projection in the textbook and/or audio-visuals. The following criteria guidelines can be used and checked as each radiograph is evaluated. (Additional checks can be placed to the left for each criteria guideline if more than six radiographs are evaluated.)

         Radiographs   Criteria Guidelines

      1 2 3 4 5 6

      __ __ __ __ __ __   a. Correct film size and correct orientation of part to film?

      __ __ __ __ __ __   b. Correct alignment and/or centering of part to film?

      __ __ __ __ __ __   c. Correct collimation and CR location?

      __ __ __ __ __ __   d. Pertinent anatomy well visualized?

      __ __ __ __ __ __   e. Motion?

      __ __ __ __ __ __   f. Optimum exposure; density and/or contrast?

      __ __ __ __ __ __   g. Patient ID information and markers?

      __ __ __ __ __ __   h. Gonadal shielding correctly placed if used?

___ 2. Based on acceptable variances to criteria factors, determine which of these radiographs are acceptable and which are unacceptable and should have been repeated.

Important: It is important that you have successfully carried out all of the exercises described above before taking the self-test and before going to your instructor for the chapter evaluation exam. If you neglect these exercises, you will not be able to meet all the objectives for this chapter and may not receive a passing grade for this course.

Answers to Review Exercise A

1. (a) right hip bone (b) left hip bone

2. (a) right hip bone (b) left hip bone (c) sacrum (d) coccyx

3. (a) innominate bone (b) os coxa

4. (a) ilium (b) ischium (c) pubis

5. Obturator foramen

6. Acetabulum

7. (a) body (b) ala (or wing)

8. (a) crest of ilium (b) anterior superior iliac spine (ASIS)

9. Ischial spine

10. (a) ilium (b) ischium

11. Ischial tuberosity

12. (a) anterior superior iliac spine (ASIS)
     (b) posterior superior iliac spine (PSIS)

13. Symphysis pubis

14. A. Support base for abdominal organs and fetus
     B. Forms birth canal

15. (a) right ischial tuberosity (b) left ischial tuberosity (c) tip of coccyx

16. Ultrasound

17. A. (a) general shape of pelvis (b) broad, shallow and more flared (c) narrower, deeper and less flared

     B. (a) angle of pubic arch (b) obtuse angle, more than ninety degrees (c) acute angle, less than ninety degrees

     C. (a) shape of pelvic inlet (b) more round in shape (c) more oval or heart shaped

18. A. (a) synovial (b) amphiarthrosis (c) none
     B. (a) synovial (b) amphiarthrosis (c) none
     C. (a) synovial (b) diarthrosis (c) ball and socket

19. Posterior and medial

20. Draw line between ASIS and symphysis pubis, go down approximately 2 1/2 inches at right angles from mid-point of this line.

21. Only 1 1/2 inches distal to mid-point of line between ASIS and symphysis pubis.

22. Should be rotated 15 to 20 degrees internally from anatomical position.

23. Lesser trochanter

Answers to Review Exercise A continued

24. A true AP hip will not visualize (or only slightly on some patients) the lesser trochanter in profile.

25. A. Sacrum
    B. Sacroiliac joint
    C. Crest of ilium
    D. ASIS, (anterior superior iliac spine)
    E. Acetabulum
    F. Obturator foramen
    G. Superior ramus of pubis
    H. Symphysis pubis
    I. Superior ramus of ischium
    J. Ischial spines
    K. Coccyx

    L. ASIS (anterior superior iliac spine)
    M. Anterior inferior iliac spine
    N. Ischial tuberosity
    O. Superior ramus of ischium
    P. Lesser sciatic notch
    Q. Ischial spine
    R. Greater sciatic notch
    S. Posterior inferior iliac spine
    T. Posterior superior iliac spine

    U. Head
    V. Fovea capitis
    W. Neck
    X. Lesser trochanter
    Y. Intertrochanteric crest
    Z. Greater trochanter

    a. Head of femur
    b. Neck
    c. Ischial tuberosity
    d. Acetabulum

26. 125

27. Lesser (only about 110 degrees)

28. (a) 15 (b) 20

29. 15-20

If you missed more than 17 blanks, you should review this section again in the textbook and/or audio-visuals before continuing.

Answers to Review Exercise B

1. A. (a) AP pelvis (b) 1 - 14 x 17 grid, crosswise (c) center of pelvis, midway between ASIS and symphysis pubis

   B. 1(a) AP pelvis | 1(b) 1 - 14 x 17 grid crosswise | 1(c) level of left femoral neck
   2(a) axiolateral of right hip | 2(b) 1 - 8 x 10 grid lengthwise

   C. 1(a) AP left hip | 1(b) 1 - 10 x 12 grid lengthwise | 1(c) level of left femoral neck
   2(a) axiolateral of left hip | 2(b) 1 - 8 x 10 grid lengthwise

   D. 1(a) AP pelvis | 1(b) 1 - 14 x 17 grid crosswise | 1(c) level of femoral heads
   2(a) bi-lateral frog-leg | 2(b) 1 - 14 x 17 grid crosswise

   E. 1(a) AP axial | 1(b) 1 - 14 x 17 grid crosswise | 1(c) CR to center of pelvis, 25° cephalad
   2(a) 25-30 degrees LPO and RPO | 2(b) 2 - 10 x 12 grids length-wise | 2(c) CR to 1 inch medial upside ASIS

2. 1-5, sacrum and coccyx, pelvic girdle and the head, neck, and greater trochanter of both femurs

3. (a) inferosuperior projection (b) Danelius-Miller method

4. Level of femoral heads, which is at upper margin of greater trochanters or 1 1/2 inches above symphysis pubis

5. A. Iliac crest
   B. Top of film slightly above crest

6. Symmetrical appearance of ilia, obturator foramina and ischial spines.

7. Equal distances from ASIS to table on both sides of patient

8. Flex and abduct both legs equally as far as possible and place plantar surfaces of both feet together.

9. An AP projection of both hips is needed for comparison

10. The left leg and foot would be rotated more externally than the right

11. The lesser trochanter would be visible in profile on the medial aspect of the left proximal femur

12. False (only uninjured hips should be rotated, rotation of injured hip could result in dislocation of the femoral head or neck at the fracture site.)

13. True (extra care however is required on females to insure that ovarian shields do not cover essential anatomy of the hips or area of interest.)

14. (a) upside (b) downside

15. A. (a) 25-30 (b) RPO or (c) LAO
    B. (a) 25-30 (b) LPO or (c) RAO

16. A. 35-40° left anterior oblique
    B. CR 12° cephalad directed to acetabulum of downside, (about 1 inch superior to level of greater trochanter and 2 inches medial to ASIS of affected side)

If you missed more than 10 blanks, you should review this section again in the textbook and/or audio-visuals before continuing.

Self-Test

My score = _____ %

Directions: Take this self-test only after completing all the review exercises and laboratory activities in this chapter. Complete directions including grading requirements are described in the front pages of this workbook and in the self-test of Chapter 1.

Test

There are 64 blanks. Each correct blank is worth 1.6 points. (Spelling is important so correct any misspellings as you grade your test.)

1. The four bones making up the pelvis are (a) _left hip_ ,
    (b) _right hip_ , (c) _sacrum_ , and (d) _coccyx_ _ilius_ .

2. The three divisions of each hip bone are (a) _ilium_ , _ileum_
    (b) _ischium_ , and (c) _pubis_ _ileus_

3. The crest of the ilium starts from an anterior landmark called the (a) _ASIS_
    and extends across the top to a posterior landmark called the (b) _PSIS_ .

4. What is the small protruding structure located directly posterior and slightly inferior to the acetabulum?
    lesser trochanter _ISCHIAL SPINE_

5. What are the two notches one directly above and one below the structure referred to in question number 4?
    A. _greater sciatic notch_
    B. _lesser sciatic notch_

6. List five important positioning landmarks involving the pelvis and hips.
    A. _crest_
    B. _ASIS_
    C. _greater trochanter_
    D. _symphysis pubis_
    E. _ischial tuberosity_

7. What is the bony part of the pelvis upon which a person sits? _ischial tuberosity_

8. What is the largest foramen in the body? _Obdurator foramen_

9. List the two divisions of the pelvic cavity and the primary function of each.

Division   Function

A. (a) _greater pelvis (false)_ (b) _hold abdominal organs_

B. (a) _lesser pelvis (true)_ (b) _birth canal_

10. The size of the triangular shaped outlet of the birth canal of the pelvis is determined by distances between three structures, the (a) _right ischial tuberosity_, (b) _left ischial tuberosity_, and (c) _tip of coccyx_.

11. Which division of the pelvis forms the actual birth canal? _lesser (true) pelvis_

12. What type of procedure or what modality is commonly used to evaluate for potential problems during the birthing process? _ultrasound_

13. Describe three structural differences between the male and female pelvis.

Male   Female

A. (a) _narrower less flared_   (b) _wider, more flared_

B. (a) _pubic arch narrower_   (b) _pubic arch wider_

C. (a) _heart shaped opening INLET_   (b) _rounded opening INLET_
a oval

14. The three joints involving the pelvis most directly are of what structural classification? _synovial_

15. What bony structure is used as a key indicator to determine sufficient internal rotation of the legs on an AP hip projection? _lesser trochanter_

16. Rotation can be detected on an AP pelvis radiograph by the asymmetrical appearance of which three structures?

A. _obdurator foramen_

B. _ischial spine_

C. _ilia (wings)_

17. If the leg and foot are in a true AP or anatomical position, the proximal femur will actually be rotated (a) _15°-20°_ degrees internally or externally? (b) _externally (?)_

18. A. In general on what type of patient (male, female, tall, short, thin, heavy) standing in the anatomical position, will the long axis of the femurs be about **10 degrees** from vertical?

male, tall, thin

B. What type will be about **15 degrees** from vertical? (Remember this difference in angle changes the amount of CR angle required on a true lateral knee projection.)

female, short, heavy

19. Describe the correct central ray location for the following:

    A. AP pelvis for hips _____ *Center of pelvis midway between level of ASIS & symphysis pubis* _____

    B. AP unilateral hip _____ *femoral neck* _____

    C. Right sacroiliac joint (posterior oblique) *LPO* _____ *1" medial to right ASIS* _____

20. In positioning a patient for an AP pelvis, how can you insure against rotation of the pelvis? _____
    distance btw. ASIS & table _____

21. Identify the two obliques, with degrees of rotation, which may be taken specifically for the **left** sacroiliac joint?

    A. Oblique? (a) *LAO* _____   Degree of rotation? (b) *30° 25°-30°* _____

    B. Oblique? (a) *RPO* _____   Degree of rotation? (b) *30° 25°-30°* _____

22. What structures are best demonstrated on an AP hip radiograph? *head & neck of* _____
    ACETABULUM, FEMORAL HEAD, NECK, GREATER TROCHANTER *femur, pelvic bones, sacrum coccyx*

23. Complete the following:

		Basic Projections		Number & Size of Film Holder(s)
A.	Unilateral hip (for poss. fracture)	1 (a) *AP pelvis (both hips for comparison)*	1(b) *14×17 grid*	
		2 (a) *axiolateral shoot-through*	2(b) *10×12 grid 8×10*	
B.	Unilateral check hip	1 (a) *AP hip (one side)*	2(b) *8×10*	
		2 (a) *axiolateral*	2(b) *8×10*	
C.	Sacroiliac joints	1 (a) *SI AP AP pelvis*	2(b) *14×17*	
		2 (a) *Obliques LPO RPO*	2(b) *10×12*	

Answers to Self-Test

1. (a) right hip bone (b) left hip bone
   (c) sacrum (d) coccyx

2. (a) ilium (b) ischium (b) pubis

3. (a) anterior superior iliac spine (ASIS)
   (b) posterior superior iliac spine (PSIS)

4. Ischial spine

5. A. Greater sciatic notch
   B. Lesser sciatic notch

6. A. Anterior superior iliac spine (ASIS)
   B. Symphysis pubis
   C. Ischial tuberosity
   D. Iliac crest
   E. Greater trochanter

7. Ischial tuberosities

8. Obturator foramen

9. A. (a) Greater or false pelvis
      (b) supports lower abdominal organs
          and fetus during pregnancy
   B. (a) Lesser or true pelvis
      (b) forms birth canal of female pelvis

10. (a) right ischial tuberosity
    (b) left ischial tuberosity
    (c) tip of coccyx

11. True pelvis

12. Ultrasound procedure

13. A. (a) Pelvis is narrower, deeper and less flared
       (b) Is broad, shallow, more flared
    B. (a) Sharper (acute) angle of pubic arch
       (b) Pubic arch relatively flat (obtuse angle)
    C. (a) Inlet is oval or heart shaped;
       (b) Inlet is nearly round

14. Synovial

15. Lesser trochanter

16. A. Ilia
    B. Ischial spines
    C. Obturator foramina

17. (a) 15 to 20 degrees (b) externally

18. A. Tall slender male patient with narrow
        pelvis
    B. Short female patient with wider pelvis

19. A. Midway between level of ASIS's and
        symphysis pubis
    B. Femoral neck
    C. One inch medial to right ASIS

20. Be sure that both ASIS's are the same distance
    from the table.

21. A. (a) RPO (b) 25-30 degrees
    B. (a) LAO (b) 25-30 degrees

22. Acetabulum, femoral head, neck, greater
    trochanter

23. A. 1(a) AP pelvis   1(b) 1-14 x 17
        2(a) Axiolateral hip   2(b) 1 - 8 x 10

    B. 1(a) AP hip   1(b) 1 - 8 x 10
        2(a) Axiolateral hip   2(b) 1 - 8 x 10

    C. 1(a) AP pelvis   1(b) 1 - 14 x 17
        2(a) 25-30 degree LPO & RPO
        2(b) 2 - 10 x 12

Chapter 8
Coccyx, Sacrum and Lumbar Spine

Rationale

The vertebral column, commonly called the spine, is an important structure radiographically and all technologists should know and understand this anatomy well. Certain projections are needed to visualize specific structures and openings of the vertebrae. The most confusing aspect of this is that different projections are required to visualize the same structures in different regions of the spine. Therefore the technologist must have a good understanding of spine anatomy and know the structural differences between various regions of the spine. The completion of this chapter should result in this type of understanding. Upon completion of this chapter you should have developed a mental image of the anatomical parts and shapes in a way that will allow you to position patients correctly to demonstrate these various structures as needed.

Recognizing various structures of a vertebra on radiographs is often difficult for technologists and the use of clearly labeled drawings followed by actual labeled radiographs in the textbook and/or audio-visuals of the same anatomical parts will help achieve this.

There are various projections which can be used to demonstrate specific parts of the spine and Part B of this chapter demonstrates these. Therefore you will learn these variations in routines and will know that if a specific routine projection cannot be taken on certain patients because of their condition or for other reasons, there are other projections which can be taken which will demonstrate the same body part just as well. Thus completion of this chapter followed by sufficient repetition on actual patients will help you become a professional technologist who can demonstrate on radiographs various parts of the vertebrae when needed.

Chapter Objectives

After you have successfully completed **all** the activities of this chapter you will be able, with at least 80% accuracy, to: (applicable to a written and/or oral examination and demonstration)

___ 1. List the five regions of the vertebral column with the correct number of vertebrae or segments in each.

___ 2. List the two primary curves of the vertebral column normally present at birth.

___ 3. List the two compensatory curves of the vertebral column which develop after birth.

___ 4. Define and describe **lordosis, kyphosis**, and **scoliosis.**

___ 5. Identify the anatomical parts of a typical vertebra on drawings, a dry skeleton and/or radiographs.

___ 6. Identify the correct medical term for a "slipped disc" and describe what causes this condition.

___ 7. Identify the two main portions of the intervertebral disc and describe their function.

___ 8. List and describe the two classifications of joints present in the vertebral column.

___ 9. Describe the condition known as spondylolisthesis.

___ 10. Identify the correct anatomical structures for the parts of the "scotty dog" demonstrated on a 45 degree oblique lumbar radiograph.

___ 11. List the basic and optional projections, size and position of film holder, central ray location, direction and degrees of angle of central ray if any, and anatomy best demonstrated on radiographic examination of the coccyx, sacrum, lumbosacral spine and L5-S1 junction.

___ 12. Position a model or articulated phantom for the projections listed above.

___ 13. Identify the correct vertebra or segment associated with the topographical landmarks of the iliac crest and the anterior superior iliac spine.

___ 14. Indicate the correct zygapophyseal joints visualized on radiographs of anterior and posterior obliques of the lumbar spine.

___ 15. Determine if the intervertebral disc spaces are "opened up" and well visualized.

___ 16. Critique and evaluate each radiograph according to evaluation criteria described in the textbook and/or audio-visuals for each projection.

___ 17. Discriminate between those radiographs which are unacceptable due to errors in positioning and incorrect exposure factors and those which are acceptable.

___ 18. Describe what the errors are on the unacceptable radiographs and explain how they could be corrected.

    (Optional if equipment is available)

___ 19. Given the necessary equipment, produce a diagnostic radiograph for the basic and optional projections of the coccyx, sacrum, lumbosacral spine, and the L5-S1 junction.

Prerequisite

The prerequisite knowledge requirement for this chapter is an understanding of radiographic terminology and the principles of exposure, radiation protection and positioning as described in Chapter 1. It is strongly suggested that a mandatory prerequisite for this chapter be the successful completion of Chapter 1.

Recommended Supplementary References

The following supplementary references, which are described in more detail in Chapter 1, are listed in a suggested order of importance and value to understanding this material.

1. *Merrill's ...,* Vol 1, pp 280-289, 330-362

2. *Clark's ...,* pp 144-180

3. *Eisenberg ...,* pp 163-167, 186-205

Learning Activity Exercises

The following review exercises should be completed only after careful study of the associated pages in the textbook and/or audio-visuals as indicated by each exercise.

After completing each of these individual exercises, check your answers with the answer sheets which follow before continuing to the next exercise.

Part I. RADIOGRAPHIC ANATOMY

Review Exercise A   The vertebral column and the anatomy of a typical vertebra, lumbar spine, sacrum and coccyx.

Textbook: pp 243-252
Audio-visuals: Unit 13, slides 1-36

1. Fill in the five regions of the vertebral column with the appropriate numbers as indicated.

		Number of Bones	
Region		Children	Adults
A. (a) _cervical_	(b) _7_	(c) _7_	
B. (a) _thoracic_	(b) _12_	(c) _12_	
C. (a) _lumbar_	(b) _5_	(c) _5_	
D. (a) _sacrum_	(b) _5_	(c) _1_	
E. (a) _coccyx_	(b) _4 (3-5)_	(c) _1_	
Total	(b) _33_	(c) _26_	

2. Which region comprises the largest of the individual vertebra? _lumbar_

3. Which two regions normally fuse into single bones in adults?

   A. _sacrum_

   B. _coccyx_

4. Which two primary curves of the vertebral column are normally present at birth?

   A. _thoracic_

   B. _sacral (pelvic)_

5. Which curve develops when a child begins to lift their head? (a) _cervical_ when they begin to walk? (b) _lumbar_

6. What is the name describing an abnormal or exaggerated lumbar curvature? _lordosis_ _concave_

7. The abnormal "hump-back" type of curvature of the thoracic region is called (a) _kyphosis_, which is (b) _convex_ (convex or concave) forward. _concave (concave)_

8. An abnormal lateral curvature is called ___Scoliosis___.

9. Fill in the following parts of a typical vertebra.:

   A.   The somewhat large process extending posteriorly from the typical vertebra is called the _____
        spinous process

   B.   The two processes extending laterally from each side of the vertebra are called transverse
        processes.

   C.   Each vertebra has four articular processes; the two above are called (a) superior
        articular processes, and the two below (b) inferior
        articular processes.

   D.   The processes in question C form an important joint when several vertebrae are stacked together
        called the zygapophyseal joint.

   E.   The articular surfaces of the processes in question C are called facets.

   F.   At the upper and lower surface of the pedicle are two notches called the (a) superior
        vertebral notch and (b) inferior vertebral notch

   G.   With several vertebrae stacked together, the two notches in question F form an important opening
        called the intervertebral foramen

   H.   The substance found between the bodies of any two vertebrae is called the inter-
        vertebral disc.

   I.   The outer fibrous portion of the answer to question H is called the (a) annulus fibrosus
        and the soft inner portion is called the (b) nucleus pulposus

   J.   What is the more common name of an HNP (herniated nucleus pulposus)? (a) slipped disc.
        This condition is caused by (b) the inner part protudes to
        press on the spinal cord or spinal nerves

10. List the (a) structural classification, and (b) mobility classification for these two joints involving the ver-
    tebral column.

    A.   Between vertebral bodies (a) cartilaginous (b) amphiorthrodial

    B.   Zygapophyseal joints (a) synovial (b) diarthrodial
         (gliding)

11. Name the labeled parts of a lumbar vertebra from these drawings.

A. pedicle

B. lamina

C. vertebral arch

D. spinous process

E. transverse process

F. facet

G. vertebral foramen

H. body

Superior View   Fig. 8-1

I. spinous process

J. superior articular process

K. transverse process

L. superior vertebral notch

M. pedicle

N. body

O. inferior vertebral notch

P. inferior articular process

Q. lamina

Lateral View   Fig 8-2

12. What is the anatomical name for the "tail bone"? ___coccyx___

13. The pointed tip of this bone is called the (a) ___apex___ , and the broader superior portion is called the (b) ___base___ .

14. There may be (a) ___3___ to ___5___ segments of this bone in children but the usual number is (b) ___4___ .

15. The forward curvature of this bone is ___more less___ (more or less) pronounced in females than in males?

16. In a young child, the sacrum has ___5___ segments which fuse into a single bone in the adult.

17. The four sets of openings on each side of the sacrum through which nerves and blood vessels pass are called ___pelvic sacral foramina___ .

18. On the posterior sacrum, the large wedge-shaped articular surface on each side is called the (a) ___auricular surface___ which is obliqued (b) ___30___ degrees backward and articulates with the pelvis at the (c) ___sacroiliac___ joint.

19. The most anterior edge of the sacrum helps to form the (a) _inlet of the true pelvis_
and is called the (b) _promontory_ .

20. The spinous processes of the sacrum are fused and form the _median sacral crest_ .

21. The small tubercles representing the inferior articular processes of the distal sacrum are called _____
sacral horns (cornua)

22. On the lumbar vertebrae, the palpable tip of each spinous process lies at the level of the _inter-_
vertebral disc space inferior to each vertebral bo

23. The last movable joint of the lower vertebral column is an important joint called the (a) _lumbo-_
sacral joint , abbreviated as the (b) _L5-S1_ joint. On a male this joint is situated at an
angle of approximately (c) _30_ degrees and on a female (d) _35_ degrees.

24. That portion of the lamina between the two articular processes may be important pathologically and
is called the _pars interarticularis_ .

25. When the part defined in question 24 fails to unite the anterior and posterior aspects of an individual
vertebra, this allows one vertebra to slip forward on the vertebral body which lies inferiorly to it. This
conditions is known as _Spondylolisthesis_ .

26. Another common deficit is caused when the two lamina fail to unite posteriorly where the spinous
process is usually found. This condition is known as a _Spina bifida_ .

27. A "scotty dog" seems to appear on a 45 degree oblique lumbar spine. Identify the various parts of the
vertebra which make up the following parts of this "scotty dog."

A. Eye   _pedicle_

B. Nose   _transverse process_

C. Ear   _Superior articular process_

D. Front leg _inferior articular process_

E. Neck   _pars interarticularis_

"Scotty Dog"   Fig. 8-3
(Oblique L. Spine)

Part II. RADIOGRAPHIC POSITIONING

Review Exercise B   Positioning of the Coccyx, Sacrum, and Lumbosacral spine

Textbook: pp 253-270
Audio-visuals: Unit 13, slides 37-72

1.   Fill in the basic projections, size and position of film cassette (LW or CW), and degrees and direction of CR angle if any. (Write in "none" if CR is not angled.)

		Basic Projections	Size & Position of Film	CR Degrees & Direction
A.	Coccyx	1(a) AP	(b) 8×10 LW	(c) 10° caudal
		2(a) lateral	(b) 8×10 LW	(c) none
B.	Sacrum	1(a) AP	(b) 10×12 LW	(c) 15° cephalic
		2(a) lateral	(b) 10×12 LW	(c) none
C.	Lumbosacral spine	1(a) AP (PA)	(b) 14×17 LW	(c) none
		2(a) Obliques	(b) 11×14 LW	(c) none
		3(a) lateral	(b) 14×17 LW	(c) none
		4(a) lat L5-S1	(b) 8×10 LW	(c) none

2.   Describe the correct lengthwise (head-to-foot) and transverse (side-to-side) centering (entrance of CR) for the following:

		Lengthwise Centering	Transverse Centering
A.	AP coccyx	(a) midsagittal plane to midline of table	(b) 2" above symphysis pubis
B.	Lateral coccyx	(a) long axis of coccyx to midline of table	(b) 1"-1½" above greater trochanter
C.	AP sacrum	(a) midsagittal plane to midline of table	(b) between symphysis pubis & ASIS
D.	Lateral sacrum	(a) long axis of sacrum to midline of table	(b) 2" anterior to posterior sacrum at level of ASIS
E.	AP or PA L spine	(a) midsagittal plane to midline of table	(b) iliac crest
F.	RPO L spine	(a) 45° rotation, spinal column at midline of table	(b) btw. iliac crest + inferior rib margin

(Continued on next page)

2. *(continued)*

		Lengthwise Centering		Transverse Centering

G. Lateral L-S spine   (a) coronal plane to midline of table   (b) iliac crest

H. AP L5-S1 junction   (a) midsagittal plane   (b) ASIS

I. Lateral L5-S1 junction   (a) 1/2" anterior from posterior surface   (b) 1 1/2" above iliac crest

3. Five important topographical landmarks are listed below. Indicate the correct vertebral level associated with these external landmarks.

A. Iliac crest ____L4 - L5____

B. ASIS ____S2____

C. Superior margin of symphysis pubis ____mid-coccyx____

D. Greater trochanter ____mid-coccyx____

E. Inferior costal margin ____L2 - L3____
(Inferior rib cage)

4. Do the exposure factors need to be **increased, decreased,** or **the same** for a lateral coccyx compared to a lateral sacrum? (a) ____decreased____. How much (if any)? (b) ____5-7 kVp____

5. On an AP lumbar spine, why should the knees and hips be flexed? ____straightens spine opens intervertebral spaces   flatten spine____

6. Two inches superior to the level of the iliac crest (which is midway between iliac crest and inferior costal margin on the **average** patient) corresponds to the level of which vertebra? ____L3 - L4____

7. On a lumbar spine, the RPO will best visualize the **right** or **left** zygapophyseal joint? ____right____

8. A 35-40° oblique best visualizes the zygapophyseal joints (scotty dogs) of the (a) ____L5-S1 L1-__ vertebrae; and the 55-60° oblique of the ____L1-L2 L5-S1____ vertebrae.

9. The LAO will visualize the same structures and give the same view as a ____RPO____.

10. Posterior obliques of the lumbar spine will best visualize the zygapophyseal joints **nearest** or **farthest** from the film? ____nearest____   RPO - right   LPO - left

11. Why is it important that the lumbar spine be near parallel to the table top on a lateral lumbosacral spine?
____straighten spine,   open intervertebral spaces____

12. List the anatomy best visualized on the following:

    A. AP lumbar spine _lumbar bodies, disc spaces, spinous + traverse processes, laminae, SI joints, sacrum_

    B. LPO of lumbar spine _left zygapophyseal joints_

    C. RAO of lumbar spine _left zygapophyseal joints_

    D. RPO of lumbar spine _right zygapophyseal joints_

    E. LAO of lumbar spine _right zygapophyseal joints_

    F. Lateral lumbosacral spine _lumbar vertebrae, intervertebral joints, spinous processes, L5-S1 junction, sacrum, first 4 intervertebral foramina_

13. A. Which angle and how many degrees is required on an AP of the L5-S1 junction ?

       (a) _cephalic_ angle, (b) _30-35_ degrees.

    B. Does this angle usually need to be **more** or **less** on a (male) than on a female? _less_

    C. If the patient's legs are flexed rather than extended, would the cephalic angle be **increased** or **decreased**? _decreased_

14. If on a lateral of the L5-S1 junction, some support was used but there was still some "sagging" of the spine, which way would the central ray be angled and approximately how many degrees?

    (a) _caudal_ , (b) _5-8_ degrees.

15. Give two significant advantages of taking a PA rather than AP for a lumbar spine on an average younger female patient.

    A. _reduces gonadal dose on females 20-30%_

    B. _opens disc spaces_

16. List four advantages of an increase in SID to 44 or 46 inches rather than 40 inches when radiographing the spine.

    A. _reduce skin dose_

    B. _reduce magnification, increase detail_

    C. _decrease anode-heel effect_

    D. _less divergence of x-ray beam_

17. List two advantages of using a relatively high kVp for scoliosis series radiographs.

    A. _more uniform density_

    B. _reduce total radiation dose_

18. Generally, where should the lower margin of the film be placed for scoliosis series radiographs?

    1" below iliac crest .

Review Exercise C   Laboratory Activity   Textbook: pp 257-270

This part of the learning activity exercise needs to be carried out in a radiographic laboratory or a general diagnostic room in a radiology department. Part B can be carried out in a classroom or any room where illuminators are available.

A.   Positioning Exercise

For this section you need another person or an articulated phantom to act as your patient. Practice the following until you can do each of them accurately and without hesitation. It is important to achieve both accuracy and speed in radiographic positioning. Place a check by each when you have achieved this.

Include the following details as you simulate the basic projections for each exam listed below:

- correct size and type of film holder
- correct location of central ray and correct centering of part to film
- correct placement of markers
- accurate collimation
- proper use of immobilizing devices when needed
- approximate correct exposure factors
- correct instructions to your patient as you simulate the exposure
- use of gonadal shields when possible

___ 1.   AP and lateral coccyx

___ 2.   AP and lateral sacrum

___ 3.   Lumbosacral spine routine (AP, lateral, obliques, lateral spot of L5-S1)

___ 4.   AP spot of L5-S1

Optional: Using either a sectional or fully articulated phantom, produce a diagnostic radiograph for each basic projection for the following:

___ 1.   AP, lateral, obliques and L5-S1 lateral spot of lumbosacral spine

___ 2.   AP and lateral coccyx

___ 3.   AP and lateral sacrum

___ 4.   AP spot of L5-S1

B.   Review of Anatomy with Radiographs

Use those radiographs provided by your instructor. (These should include acceptable quality radiographs of the coccyx, sacrum and lumbosacral spine.)

___ 1.   Examine radiographs of the coccyx, sacrum and lumbosacral spine and identify all those anatomical parts described and demonstrated in the textbook and/or audio-visuals.

C. Film Critique and Evaluation

Your instructor will provide various radiographs of the coccyx, sacrum and lumbosacral spine for these exercises. Some will be optimal quality radiographs meeting all or most of the evaluation criteria described for each projection in the textbook and/or audio-visuals. Others will be less than optimal quality and several will be unacceptable, requiring a repeat exam. You should evaluate each radiograph as specified below.

Place a check by each of the following when it is completed.

__ 1.   Critique each radiograph based on evaluation criteria provided for each projection in the textbook and/or audio-visuals. The following criteria guidelines can be used and checked as each radiograph is evaluated. (Additional checks can be placed to the left for each criteria guideline if more than six radiographs are evaluated.)

Radiographs	Criteria Guidelines
1 2 3 4 5 6	

__ __ __ __ __ __   a. Correct film size and correct orientation of part to film?

__ __ __ __ __ __   b. Correct alignment and/or centering of part to film?

__ __ __ __ __ __   c. Correct collimation and CR location?

__ __ __ __ __ __   d. Pertinent anatomy well visualized?

__ __ __ __ __ __   e. Motion?

__ __ __ __ __ __   f. Optimum exposure; density and/or contrast?

__ __ __ __ __ __   g. Patient ID information and markers?

__ 2.   Based on acceptable variances to criteria factors, determine which of these radiographs are acceptable and which are unacceptable and should have been repeated.

IMPORTANT: It is important that you have successfully carried out all of the exercises described above before taking the self-test and before going to your instructor for the chapter evaluation exam. If you neglect these exercises, you will not be able to meet all objectives for this chapter and may not receive a passing grade for this course.

Answers to Review Exercise A

1. A.   (a) Cervical   (b) 7   (c) 7
    B.   (a) Thoracic   (b) 12   (c) 12
    C.   (a) Lumbar   (b) 5   (c) 5
    D.   (a) Sacrum   (b) 5   (c) 1
    E.   (a) Coccyx   (b) 4 (3-5) (c) 1
    Total   (b) 33   (c) 26

2. Lumbar

3. A.   Sacrum
    B.   Coccyx

4. A.   Thoracic
    B.   Sacral

5. (a) cervical curve
    (b) lumbar curve

6. lordosis

7. (a) kyphosis (b) concave

8. scoliosis

9. A.   spinous process
    B.   transverse processes
    C.   (a) superior articular processes (b) inferior articular processes
    D.   zygapophyseal
    E.   facets
    F.   (a) superior vertebral notch (b) inferior vertebral notch
    G.   intervertebral foramen
    H.   intervertebral disc
    I.   (a) annulus fibrosus (b) nucleus pulposus
    J.   (a) slipped disc
          (b) the nucleus pulposus protruding, through injury, to press on the spinal chord or nerve roots

10. A.   (a) cartilaginous (b) amphiarthrodial
    B.   (a) synovial (b) diarthrodial

11. A.   Pedicle
    B.   Lamina
    C.   Vertebral arch
    D.   Spinous process
    E.   Transverse process
    F.   Facet of superior articular process
    G.   Vertebral foramen
    H.   Body

    I.   Spinous process
    J.   Superior articular process
    K.   Transverse process
    L.   Superior vertebral notch
    M.   Pedicle
    N.   Body
    O.   Inferior vertebral notch
    P.   Inferior articular process (facet)
    Q.   Lamina

Answers to Review Exercise A continued

12.   Coccyx

13.   (a) apex   (b) base

14.   (a) 3 to 5   (b) 4

15.   less

16.   5

17.   pelvic (anterior) sacral foramina

18.   (a) auricular surface   (b) 30   (c) sacroiliac

19.   (a) inlet of true pelvis   (b) promontory

20.   median sacral crest

21.   sacral horns

22.   intervertebral disc space inferior to the body of that vertebra

23.   (a) lumbosacral joint   (b) L5-S1   (c) 30   (d) 35

24.   pars interarticularis

25.   spondylolisthesis

26.   spina bifida

27.   A.   Pedicle
           B.   Transverse process
           C.   Superior articular process
           D.   Inferior articular process
           E.   Pars interarticularis

If you missed more than 18 blanks, you should review this section again in the textbook and/or **audio-visuals** before continuing.

Answers to Review Exercise B

1. A. 1(a) AP   (b) 8 x 10 LW   (c) 10   Caudal
      2(a) Lateral   (b) 8 x 10 LW   (c) None

    B. 1(a) AP   (b) 10 x 12 LW   (c) 15   Cephalad
      2(a) Lateral   (b) 10 x 12 LW   (c) None

    C. 1(a) AP   (b) 14 x 17 LW   (c) None
      2(a) Lateral   (b) 14 x 17 LW   (c) None
      3(a) R & L obliques   (b) 11 x 14 LW (or 10 x 12)   (c) None
      4(a) L5, S1 lateral   (b) 8 x 10 LW   (c) None (with proper support)

2. A. (a) 2" (5 cm) superior to symphysis pubis   (b) Midsagittal plane
    B. (a) 1/2" (1 cm) superior to level of greater trochanter   (b) Coccyx to midline of table
    C. (a) Midway between symphysis pubis and the ASIS's   (b) Midsagittal plane
    D. (a) Level of ASIS   (b) ~2" (5 cm) anterior to posterior sacrum
    E. (a) Level of iliac crest, or 1 1/2 inches above iliac crest with 11 x 14 film
        (b) Midsagittal plane
    F. (a) Midway between iliac crest and inferior rib margin (L3 level or L3-L4 disc space)
        (b) 2" (5 cm) anterior to spinous process of L3
    G. (a) Level of iliac crest , or 1 1/2 inches above iliac crest with 11 x 14 film
        (b) Coronal plane to midline of table
    H. (a) Level of ASIS   (b) Midsagittal plane
    I. (a) 1 1/2" inferior to iliac crests   (b) 1 1/2" anterior from posterior surface

3. A. L4-L5 disc space
    B. 2nd sacral segment
    C. Mid coccyx
    D. Mid coccyx
    E. L2 (or L2-L3 disc space)

4. (a) Decrease   (b) 5-7 kVp

5. Will reduce lordotic curvature (flatten out spine)

6. L3 or L3-L4 disc space

7. Right

8. (a) L1-L2 (proximal lumbar vertebrae)   (b) L5-S1(distal lumbar vertebrae)

9. RPO

10. Nearest

11. The disc spaces will not be opened if the spine is not parallel

12. A. Lumbar bodies and their disc spaces, spinous and transverse processes, the laminae, SI joints and
       sacrum
    B. Left zygapophyseal joints
    C. Left zygapophyseal joints
    D. Right zygapophyseal joints
    E. Right zygapophyseal joints
    F. Lumbar vertebrae and intervertebral joints, spinous processes, L5-S1 junction, sacrum and first four
       intervertebral foramina.

Answers to Review Exercise B continued

13. A. (a) cephalad   (b) 30-35 degrees
     B. Less
     C. Decreased

14. (a) Caudal   (b) approximately 5 to 8 degrees

15. A. Reduces gonadal dose on females by 20-30%
     B. Places the natural curvature of L spine nearer parallel to divergent x-ray beam
         (Opens disc spaces better)

16. A. Reduces skin dose
     B. Reduces magnification and increases detail
     C. Decrease in the anode-heel effect
     D. Facilitates "opening up" intervertebral spaces by less divergence of x-ray beam
         (If spine is parallel to film)

17. A. Longer scale contrast therefore more uniform density between thoracic and lumbar vertebrae.
     B. Reduction in total radiation dose to patients (usually younger patients requiring repeat exams over a
         period of time)

18. 1 inch below iliac crest

If you missed more than 25 blanks, you should review this section again in the textbook and/or audio-visuals before continuing.

Self-Test

My score = _____ %

Directions: Take this self-test only after completing all the review exercises and laboratory activities in this chapter. Complete directions including grading requirements are described in the front pages of this workbook and in the self-test of Chapter 1.

Test

There are 72 blanks. Each correct blank is worth approximately 1.4 points. (Spelling is important so correct any misspellings as you grade your test.)

1. Define the following terms:

    A. Scoliosis _lateral curvature_

    B. Lordosis _extreme (abnormal) lumbar curve   concave_

    C. Kyphosis _hump-back - extreme thoracic curve (abnormal) (convex)_

2. What parts of the vertebrae form the zygapophyseal joints? _superior + inferior articular processes_

3. What parts of the vertebrae make up the intervertebral foramen? _superior + inferior vertebral notch_

4. What is the term describing the articular surfaces of the zygapophyseal joints? _facets_

5. What are the four parts of a vertebra which make up the vertebral arch?

    A. Two _pedicles_

    B. Two _lamina_

6. What is the name of the opening formed by the body in front and the vertebral arch laterally and posteriorly? _intervertebral foramen_

7. What is the name of the long tubular shaped opening extending along the complete length of the spine formed by a succession of the openings described in question 6? _Spinal canal (column)_

8. What is the inner soft portion of the intervertebral disc called? _nucleus pulposas_

9. What are the initials and the medical term for a "slipped disc?" (a) Initials _HNP_
    (b) Medical term _herniated nucleus pulposus_

annulus fibrosus

10. What causes the condition identified in question 9? _inner part of disc pushing out to spinal cord or nerve roots_

11. In children there are (a) _5_ sacral segments and (b) _3-5_ coccygeal segments.

12. In adults there are (a) _26_ separate bones making up the spinal column, and in children there are usually (b) _33_ .

13. The typical vertebra has two bony processes extending laterally called (a) _transverse processe_, and one process extending posteriorly called the (b) _spinous process_ .

14. The typical vertebra has four articular processes; the two above are called (a) _superior_ _____ and the two below are (b) _inferior_ .

15. A. What is the structural classification of joints formed by the processes in question 14? _synovial_ .

    B. What is the mobility classification of these joints ? _diarthrodial_

    C. What is the movement type? _gliding_

16. A. What structures make up the second type of joint in the vertebral column ? _intervertebral_ _bodies of verteb_

    B. What is the structural classification? _cartilagenous_   _joints_

    C. What is the mobility classification? _amphiarthrodial_

17. What are the four possible movements of the total vertebral column?

    A. _flexion_

    B. _extension_

    C. _lateral flexion_

    D. _rotation_

18. The pointed tip of the coccyx is the (a) _apex_ and the broader superior portion is the (b) _base_ .

19. The four sets of holes on the sacrum which transmit nerves and blood vessels are called (a) _anterior sacral foramina_ on the anterior and (b) _posterior sacral forami_ on the posterior.

20. The large masses of bone lateral to the first segment of the sacrum are called _ala or wings_

21. The anterior border of the body of the first segment of the sacrum is called the _promontory_ .

22. The L5-S1 joint forms an angle of approximately (a) _30-35°_ degrees; this angle is (b) _lesser_ (greater or lesser) on females than on males? _greater_

23. Describe that portion of the vertebra which is called the pars interarticularis. *Central portion of lamina between inferior & superior articular processes*

24. Describe the condition of spondylolisthesis. *one vertebra slips forward on the vertebral body below it*

25. Describe the condition of spina bifida. *two lamina fail to unite leaving an opening where the spinous process should be*

26. The condition described in question 25 most often occurs at which vertebra? *L5.*

27. Identify the parts of a "scotty dog" appearing on an oblique lumbar spine.

    A.   The pars interarticularis appears as the ____*neck*____ part of the scotty dog.

    B.   The transverse process appears as the ___*nose*___.

    C.   The pedicle appears as the ____*eye*____.

    D.   The superior articular process appears as the *ear*.

    E.   The inferior articular process appears as the *front leg*.

28. Identify the correct vertebra or segment corresponding to the following on an average patient:

    A.   ASIS *2nd sacral segment   2S*

    B.   Iliac crest *L4-L5 disk space*

    C.   2 inches superior to iliac crest *L3 or L3-L4 disc space*

    D.   Greater trochanter *mid coccyx*

    E.   Lower costal (rib) margin *L2 or L2·L3 disc space*

29. The LPO of the lumbar spine visualizes the ___*left*___ (right or left) zygapophyseal joints.
    RAO   RPO, LAO = right
30. Which anterior oblique will visualize the same structures as an LPO? *RAO*

31. Fill in the degrees and direction of CR angle for the following:

    A.   AP L5-S1 junction   *30-35*   degrees *cephalic*

    B.   AP coccyx   *10*   degrees *caudal*

    C.   AP sacrum   *15*   degrees *cephalic*

32. The medial sacral crest of the sacrum on an adult is made up of certain bones which become fused. These are the *fused spinous processes of sacrum*.

33. The sacral horns represent the *inferior articular processes* which project down on each side of the fifth sacral segment.

34. List two advantages of taking lumbosacral radiographs as PA projections rather than AP.

    A. _less radiation to gonadal area of females_

    B. _opens disc spaces_

35. List three advantages of using an increased SID for radiographing the spine.

    A. _less magnification, more detail_

    B. _reduced skin dosage_

    C. _opens disc space_　　　_reduces anode-heel effec_

36. A (a) _35-40_ degree oblique best visualizes the zygapophyseal joints of L1-L2 , and (b) _55-60_

    degree oblique for visualizing the L5-S1 region.

Answers to Self-Test

1. A. Abnormal lateral spinal curvature
   B. An abnormal or exaggerated lumbar curvature
   C. An abnormal thoracic "hump-back" type of curvature

2. Superior articular processes of one vertebra with inferior articular processes of another

3. Inferior vertebral notch of one vertebra with superior vertebral notch of another

4. Facets

5. A. Pedicles
   B. Laminae

6. Vertebral foramen

7. Spinal canal

8. Nucleus pulposus

9. (a) HNP
   (b) herniated nucleus pulposus

10. The nucleus pulposus, protruding through injury, presses on the spinal cord or nerve roots.

11. (a) 5 (b) 3-5 (4)

12. (a) 26 (b) 33

13. (a) transverse processes
    (b) spinous processes

14. (a) superior articular processes
    (b) inferior articular processes

15. A. Synovial joints
    B. Diarthrodial (freely movable)
    C. Gliding

16. A. Bodies of vertebra (intervertebral joint)
    B. Cartilaginous
    C. Amphiarthrodial

17. A. Flexion
    B. Extension
    C. Lateral flexion (bending)
    D. Rotation

18. (a) apex (b) base

19. (a) anterior sacral foramina
    (b) posterior sacral foramina

20. Alae (or wings)

21. Promontory

22. (a) 30-35 (b) greater

23. That central portion of the lamina which lies between the inferior and superior articular processes.

24. One vertebra slips forward on the vertebral body below it.

25. When the two laminae fail to unite, leaving an opening where the spinous process is usually found

26. L5

27. A. Neck
    B. Nose
    C. Eye
    D. Ear
    E. Front leg

28. A. 2nd sacral segment
    B. L4-L5 disc space
    C. L3, or L3-L4 disc space
    D. Mid coccyx
    E. L2, or L2-L3 disc space

29. Left

30. Right (RAO)

31. A. 30-35 Cephalad
    B. 10 Caudal
    C. 15 Cephalad

32. Fused spinous processes of sacral segments

33. Inferior articular processes

34. A. Reduces gonadal exposure on females
    B. Opens disc spaces better

35. A. Reduced skin dose
    B. Reduces magnification and increases detail
    C. Reduces anode-heel effect
    or 4th option:
    Opens disc spaces better on laterals if spine is parallel to film

36. (a) 35-40 (b) 55-60

Chapter 9
Thoracic and Cervical Spine

Rationale

The importance of the vertebral column including the structures protected by these various bones was discussed in the preceding chapter. However, the importance of a thorough understanding of the anatomy of the vertebral column cannot be overemphasized. Only when you possess a complete knowledge of the similarities and differences of the entire spine will you be able to produce quality radiographs on any part of this important area. After the completion of this chapter, you should possess a working knowledge of the anatomy and positioning of the total vertebral column.

You will be able to determine the specific anatomy best shown on each projection or position of each section of the vertebral column. Occasionally individual vertebrae must be radiographed. A list of various topographical landmarks will be given to enable you to locate any specific vertebra with the precision necessary.

Suggested standard routines with the more common optional projections will again be presented. In some cases, alternative methods to achieve the end result will be given for use on the patient who cannot assume the recommended position. You should be able to, at the completion of this chapter and followed by sufficient repetition on actual patients, produce quality radiographs of any part or section of the cervical and thoracic regions of the vertebral column.

Chapter Objectives

After you have successfully completed **all** the activities of this chapter, you will be able, with at least 80% accuracy, to: (applicable to a written and/or oral examination and demonstration)

___ 1. Identify, on drawings, radiographs, and on a skeleton all anatomy of the thoracic and cervical spine as described in the textbook and/or audio-visuals.

___ 2. Identify those features of the thoracic and cervical vertebrae which distinguish them from any other region.

___ 3. Locate on an articulated skeleton, any costovertebral or costotransverse joint.

___ 4. List one additional name for C1, C2, and C7.

___ 5. Locate any specific vertebra from C1 to the coccyx by using other palpable bony landmarks.

___ 6. Determine which position or projection of each section of the spine will best demonstrate zygapophyseal joints or intervertebral foramina, and whether the right or left side is being visualized.

___ 7. List the basic and optional projections, size and type of film holder, central ray location, direction and angulation of the central ray, if necessary, and anatomy best demonstrated on radiographic examination of the thoracic and cervical spine.

___ 8. Position a model or articulated phantom, to demonstrate the basic and optional projections as given in the textbook and/or audio-visuals for thoracic and cervical spines.

Given several radiographs of the thoracic and cervical spines to view:

___   9.   Critique and evaluate each radiograph according to evaluation criteria described in the textbook and/or audio-visuals.

___   10.   Discriminate between radiographs which are acceptable and those which are unacceptable because of exposure factors, collimation, or overall lack of positioning accuracy.

___   11.   Describe how any positioning or technical error could be corrected to produce a satisfactory result.

Optional if equipment is available:

___   12   Given the necessary equipment, and an articulated or sectional phantom, produce a diagnostic radiograph for the basic and optional projections of the thoracic and cervical spine.

Prerequisite

The prerequisite knowledge requirement for this chapter is an understanding of radiographic terminology and the principles of exposure, radiation protection and positioning as described in Chapter 1. It is strongly suggested that a mandatory prerequisite for this chapter be the successful completion of Chapter 1.

Recommended Supplementary References

The following supplementary references, which are described in more detail in Chapter 1, are listed in a suggested order of importance and value to understanding this material.

1.   *Merrill's ...*, Vol 1, pp 282-329

2.   *Clark's ...*, pp 148-165

3.   *Eisenberg ...*, pp 168-187

Learning Exercises

The following review exercises should be completed only after careful study of the associated pages in the textbook and/or audio-visuals as indicated by each exercise.

After completing each of these individual exercises, check your answers with the answer sheets which follow before continuing to the next exercise.

Part I. RADIOGRAPHIC ANATOMY

Review Exercise A   Anatomy of Thoracic and Cervical Spine   Textbook: pp 271-279
Audio-visuals, unit 14, slides 1-36

1. What is the one feature of all thoracic vertebrae which makes them different from all other vertebrae?
    Facets for rib articulations

2. A. Identify those thoracic vertebra(e) having full facets. _I1, T10-T12 T11, T12_
    B. Identify those thoracic vertebra(e) having two demifacets on each side. _T2-T9 T1-T10_

3. The costotransverse joints are between the (a) _tubercles_ of each rib and the (b) _____
    transverse processes of the thoracic vertebrae, and are present on thoracic vertebrae (c) T_1_
    to T_10_.

4. The costovertebral joints are between the (a) _head_ of each rib and the
    (b) _facets or demifacets_ of thoracic vertebrae and are present on
    (c) T_1_ to T_12_ vertebrae.

5. How does the spinous process of a thoracic vertebra differ from a typical lumbar vertebra? _____
    longer and points more downward

6. Identify the parts of typical thoracic vertebrae on the following drawings:

    A. _Spinous process_
    B. _inferior articular process_
    C. _transverse process_
    D. _superior articular process_
    E. _zygapophyseal joint_
    F. _body_
    G. _intervertebral foramen_

Thoracic Vertebrae   Fig. 9-1
(Lateral View)

183

6. *(continued)*

T11-T12 facets
T1-T10 demifacets

H. <u>facet for head of rib</u>

I. <u>pedicle</u>

J. <u>facet of superior articular process</u>

K. <u>facet of transverse process</u>

L. <u>lamina</u>

M. <u>spinous process</u>

N. <u>costotransverse joint</u>

O. <u>rib</u>

P. <u>costovertebral joint</u>

Q. <u>body</u>

Posterior

Anterior

Thoracic Vertebra
(Superior View)   Fig. 9-2

7. A. What is the anatomical name for C1? <u>atlas</u>

    B. What is the anatomical name for C2? <u>axis</u>

8. Much of the rotation of the head occurs between C<u>1</u> and C<u>2</u> which helps in describing the anatomical name for one of the vertebrae in question 7.

9. (a) C<u>7</u> has many of the features of a thoracic vertebra including an extra long spinous process which gives it the special anatomical name, the (b) <u>vertebra prominens</u>.

10. The transverse process of a typical cervical vertebra is smaller than a typical lumbar vertebra and also has a hole in it called the <u>transverse foramen</u>.

11. The spinous process is shorter and on some of the cervical vertebrae ends in two projections. This double ended spinous process is said to have a <u>bifid</u> tip.

12. Describe the area called the articular pillar on a typical cervical vertebra. <u>Column of bone behind transverse process at junction of pedicle + lamina</u>

13. Located on top of this pillar is the (a) <u>superior articular process</u>, and on the bottom is the (b) <u>inferior articular process</u>

14. What is the one major distinctive feature of all cervical vertebrae? <u>transverse foramen</u>

15. Identify the parts of a typical cervical vertebra as labeled on these drawings:

A. articular pillar

B. superior articular process

C. body

D. inferior articular process

E. spinous process

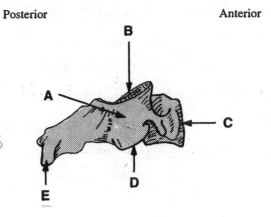

Cervical Vertebra   Fig. 9-3
(Lateral View)

F. spinous process

G. superior articular process

H. transverse foramen

I. body

J. transverse process

K. pedicle

L. lamina

M. vertebral foramen

N. bifid tip

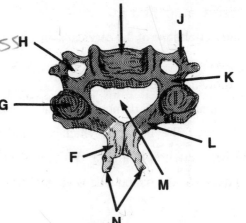

Cervical Vertebra   Fig. 9-4
(Superior View)

16. The important distinctive feature of C2 is the presence of a process of bone projecting from the upper surface of the body called the (a) __dens__, sometimes also called the (b)_____ odontoid process

17. C1 has no body but simply an arch of bone at the front called the (a) anterior arch .
Embryologically the body of C1 has fused to C2 and is called the (b) __dens__ ,
which acts as a pivot for rotation of the head.   odontoid process

18. Identify the labeled parts and the vertebra on this frontal open-mouth view of C1 and C2.

    A. _Superior articular process of C2_
    B. _transverse process of C1_
    C. _dens (odontoid process)_
    D. _lateral mass of C1_
    E. _inferior articular surface of C1_
    F. _zygapophyseal joint space_
    G. _body of C2_

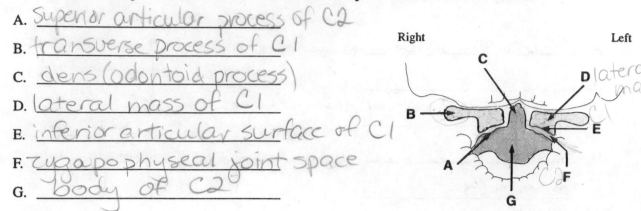

Fig. 9-5

19. The zygapophyseal joints and the intervertebral foramina are important areas radiographically. Which of these is demonstrated on a lateral cervical? (a) _zygapophyseal joints_

    On a 45° oblique? (b) _intervertebral foramen_.

20. The left anterior oblique (LAO) will demonstrate the same structures as a _right_ posterior oblique.

21. In a posterior oblique position of the cervical spine, which intervertebral foramina will be opened, the side **closest** or **farthest** from the film? _farthest_

22. In an anterior oblique of the cervical spine, which side will be opened, the **closest** or **farthest** from the film? _closest_

23. On the thoracic spine, the (a) _lateral_ position (oblique or lateral) demonstrates the interverte-bral foramina. Which demonstrates the zygapophyseal joints? (b) _70° oblique_

24. Complete the following chart which summarizes the positions best visualizing the zygapophyseal joints and the intervertebral foramina. Write in the correct answers. If the answer is an oblique, write in the correct degrees, and which side is visualized on a posterior oblique, the upside or downside.

	1. Cervical	2. Thoracic	3. Lumbar
A. Intervertebral foramina Obli. or lat. -	1(a) _oblique_	2(a) _lateral_	3(a) _lateral_
Degrees -	1(b) _45°_ °	2(b) _____ °	3(b) _____ °
Posterior Oblique - Upside or Downside -	1(c) _upside_ LPO RPO	2(c) _____	3(c) _____
B. Zygapophyseal Obli. or lat. -	1(a) _lateral_	2(a) _oblique_	3(a) _oblique_
Degrees -	1(b) _____ °	2(b) _70_ °	3(b) _45°_ °
Posterior Oblique - Upside or Downside -	1(c) _____	2(c) _upside_ LPO RPO	3(c) _downside_ LPO RPO

Part II. RADIOGRAPHIC POSITIONING

Review Exercise B   Topographical Landmarks and Positioning of Thoracic and Cervical Spine

Textbook: pp 280-295
Audio-visuals, Unit 14, slides 37-72

1. Name the following main parts of the sternum and associated topographical landmarks.

   A. Upper portion of bone _manubrium_

   B. Superior margin of this upper section _suprasternal notch (jugular notch)_

   C. Main center portion of sternum _body_

   D. Area of joint between top and center portions _sternal angle_

   E. Most inferior aspect of sternum _xiphoid tip_

2. Identify the correct vertebrae corresponding to the following topographical landmarks on an average erect male.

   1" above C1, EAM
   C1 mastoid tip

   A. Sternal angle _T4-T5_   _T4-5_   _C3 gonion (angle of jaw)_

   B. Jugular notch _T2-T3_   _T2-3_   _(C4-C6) C5 thyroid cartilage_

   C. 3-4 inches below jugular notch _T7_   _T7_   _C7 vertebra prominens (T1)_

   D. 1-2 inches above jugular notch _T1_   _T1_   _T1 1-2" above jugular notch_

   E. Xiphoid tip _T10_   _T10_   _T2-T3 jugular notch_

   F. Vertebra prominens _C7/T1_   _C7-T1_   _T4-T5 sternal angle_

   G. Thyroid cartilage _C5 (C4-C6)_   _2-3_   _T7 3-4" below jugular notch (aug center of chest)_

   H. Gonion (angle of jaw) _C3_   _C3_   _T10 xiphoid tip_

   I. Mastoid tip _C1_   _C1_   _L2-L3 lower costal margin_

   C4-L5 iliac crest

   J. EAM (external acoustic meatus) _1" above C1_   _1" above C1_   _S2 ASIS_   _C4-T3_
   lower cervical

3. The swimmer's position is used to demonstrate what region of the spine? _upper thoracic_

4. What is the purpose of the breathing technique on a lateral thoracic projection? _blurring of ribs & lung markings_

5. Fill in the anatomy best demonstrated on the following projections:

   A. LPO of thoracic spine _upside (right) zygapophyseal joints_

   B. RAO of thoracic spine _downside (right) zygapophyseal joints_

5. *(continued)*

C. AP cervical _C3-C7, vertebral bodies, space between_
    pedicles, intervertebral disc spaces, spinous process

D. LAO of cervical spine _intervertebral foramen - downside_ (left)

E. RPO of cervical SPINE _upside intervertebral foramen_ left

F. Open mouth AP cervical _odontoid process (dens), C-2 body,_
    C1 lateral masses, zygapophyseal joints

6. Describe the correct central ray location for the following and indicate direction and degrees of CR angle where applicable.

		CR location	Direction and degrees of angle of CR
A.	AP & lateral thoracic spine	(a) _CR to T7 3-4" below jugular notch_	
B.	Swimmer's lateral	(a) _CR to T1, 1½" above jugular notch_ C7-T1	
C.	AP cervical	(a) _C5-C6 (lower margin of thyroid cartilage)_	(b) _15°-20° cepha_
D.	Posterior obli. cervical (AP projection) LPO RPO	(a) _C4 - upper margin of thyroid cartilage_	(b) _15°-20° cephal_
E.	Anterior obli. cervical (PA projection) LAO RAO	(a) _C4- upper margin of thyroid cartilage_	(b) _15°-20° cauda_

7. On a patient with a severe neck injury, which projection should always be taken first? (a) _lateral cervical horizontal beam_ Why is this? (b) _to check for cervical or skull trauma_

8. Why should the lateral cervical spine be taken at 72 inches SID? _large OID - compensates for loss of image sharpness • magnifica_

9. The lateral cervical spine should be taken on **inhalation** or **exhalation**? (a) _exhalation_
    Why? (b) _maximum shoulder depression_

10. A. To insure visualization of certain key anatomical structures, what is the one most important positioning step for the cervical AP open mouth projection? _proper tilt of head_

    B. Why is this so important? _teeth or skull will superimpose_

Review Exercise C   Laboratory Activity   Textbook: pp 280-295

This part of the learning activity exercise needs to be carried out in a radiographic laboratory or a general diagnostic room in a radiology department. Part B can be carried out in a classroom or any room where illuminators are available.

A. Positioning Exercise

For this section you need another person to act as your patient. Practice the following until you can do each of them accurately and without hesitation. It is important to achieve both accuracy and speed in radiographic positioning. Place a check by each when you have achieved this.
Include the following details as you simulate the basic projections for each exam listed below:

  - correct size and type of film holder
  - correct location of central ray and correct centering of part to film
  - correct placement of markers
  - accurate collimation
  - proper use of immobilizing devices when needed
  - approximate correct exposure factors
  - correct instructions to your patient as you simulate the exposure
  - gonadal shielding as necessary

___ 1. AP and lateral thoracic spine

___ 2. 70° oblique thoracic spine

___ 3. Cervical spine routine (AP, both obliques, and lateral)

___ 4. Crosstable lateral cervical

___ 5. AP open-mouth of C1 and C2

___ 6. AP cervical (moving jaw)

___ 7. Swimmer's lateral of cervicothoracic region

Optional

Using either a sectional or fully articulated phantom, produce a diagnostic radiograph for each of the following:

___ 1. AP and lateral spine

___ 2. 70° oblique thoracic spine

B. Review of Anatomy

Use those radiographs provided by your instructor.

1. Examine radiographs of the thoracic and cervical spine and identify all anatomical parts as described in the textbook and/or audiovisuals.

2. Locate bony landmarks on the radiographs and determine which vertebrae are at the levels of which landmarks.

C. Film Critique and Evaluation

Your instructor will provide radiographs of the thoracic and cervical spine for these exercises. Some will be optimal quality meeting all or nearly all evaluation criteria as described in the textbook and/or audio-visuals. Others will be less than optimal, and several will be unacceptable requiring repeat exams. You should critique or evaluate each radiograph carefully and individually following the steps below.

___ 1. Critique each radiograph based on evaluation criteria provided for each projection in the textbook and/or audio-visuals. The following criteria guidelines can be used and checked as each radiograph is evaluated.

Radiographs	Criteria Guidelines
1 2 3 4 5 6	

___ ___ ___ ___ ___ ___   a. Correct film size and correct orientation of part to film?

___ ___ ___ ___ ___ ___   b. Correct alignment and/or centering of part to film or portion of film being used?

___ ___ ___ ___ ___ ___   c. Correct collimation and CR location?

___ ___ ___ ___ ___ ___   d. Pertinent anatomy well visualized?

___ ___ ___ ___ ___ ___   e. Motion?

___ ___ ___ ___ ___ ___   f. Optimum exposure; density and/or contrast?

___ ___ ___ ___ ___ ___   g. Patient ID information and markers?

___ 2. Based on acceptable variances to criteria factors, determine which of these radiographs are acceptable and which are unacceptable and should have been repeated.

___ 3. Evaluate sufficient open-mouth dens view radiographs to determine if the base of the skull or the maxillary teeth are overlying the dens. Determine if, by tilting the head differently, the dens could be better visualized.

Important: It is important that you have successfully carried out all of the exercises described above before taking the self-test and before going to your instructor for the chapter evaluation exam. If you neglect these exercises, you will not be able to meet all the objectives for this chapter and may not receive a passing grade for this course.

Answers to Review Exercise A

1. Every thoracic vertebra has facets for articulation with ribs.

2. A. T11 & 12
   B. T1-10

3. (a) Tubercle
   (b) Transverse process
   (c) 1, 10

4. (a) Head
   (b) Facets or demifacets of the body
   (c) 1, 12

5. Thoracic vertebra spinous process is longer and points more downward.

6. A. Spinous process
   B. Inferior articular process
   C. Transverse process
   D. Superior articular process
   E. Zygapophyseal joint
   F. Body
   G. Intervertebral foramen

   H. Facet for head of rib
   I. Pedicle
   J. Facet of superior articular process
   K. Facet of transverse process
   L. Lamina
   M. Spinous process
   N. Costotransverse joint
   O. Rib
   P. Costovertebral joint
   Q. Body

7. A. Atlas
   B. Axis

8. 1 and 2

9. (a) 7 (b) vertebra prominens

10. Transverse foramen

11. Bifid

12. The short column of bone at the junction of the pedicle and lamina.

13. (a) Superior articular process
    (b) Inferior articular process

14. All have transverse foramina.

15. A. Articular pillar (pillar)
    B. Superior articular process
    C. Body
    D. Inferior articular process
    E. Spinous process

    F. Spinous process
    G. Superior articular process
    H. Transverse foramen
    I. Body
    J. Transverse process
    K. Pedicle (floor of intervertebral foramen)
    L. Lamina
    M. Vertebral foramen
    N. Bifid tip

16. (a) Dens (b) Odontoid process

17. (a) Anterior arch   (b) Dens

18. A. Superior articular surface of C2
    B. Transverse process of C1
    C. Dens (odontoid process) of C2
    D. Lateral mass of C1
    E. Inferior articular surface of C1
    F. Zygapophyseal joint space between C1 & C2
    G. Body of C2

19. (a) Zygapophyseal joints
    (b) Intervertebral foramina

20. Right (RPO)

21. Farthest

22. Closest

23. (a) Lateral
    (b) Oblique

24. A. 1(a) Obli.   2(a) Lat.   3(a) Lat.
       1(b) 45   2(b) -   3(b) -
       1(c) Upside 2(c) -   3(c) -

    B. 1(a) Lat.   2(a) Obli. 3(a) Obli.
       1(b) -   2(b) 70   3(b) 45
       1(c) -   2(c) Upside 3(c) Downside

Answers to Review Exercise B

1. A. Manubrium
   B. Jugular notch
   C. Body
   D. Sternal angle
   E. Xiphoid process

2. A. T4-T5
   B. T2-T3
   C. T7
   D. T1
   E. T10
   F. T1
   G. C5 (C4-6)
   H. C3
   I. C1
   J. 1 inch above C1

3. Cervicothoracic region C4-T3

4. To "blur out" ribs and lung tissue to better visualize thoracic vertebrae.

5. A. Right zygapophyseal joints
   B. Right zygapophyseal joints
   C. The lower 3 to 7 cervical bodies, intervertebral spaces, space between pedicles and spinous processes.
   D. Left intervertebral foramina (downside)
   E. Left intervertebral foramina (upside)
   F. Dens (odontoid process) of C2, lateral masses of C1, vertebral body of C2, and the zygapophyseal joints between C1 and C2.

6. A. (a) T7 (3-4 inches below jugular notch or 1-2 inches below sternal angle)
   B. (a) T1 (1 1/2 inches above jugular notch or at level of vertebra prominens posteriorly)
   C. (a) Enter at C5-C6 (lower margin of thyroid cartilage) (b) 15-20° cephalad
   D. (a) C4 (upper margin of thyroid cartilage) (b) 15-20° cephalad
   E. (a) C4 (b) 15-20° caudal

7. (a) Crosstable lateral
   (b) To check for possible fractures to the cervical area before moving patient for cervical routine

8. To compensate for increased OID (decreases magnification and increases detail)

9. (a) Exhalation
   (b) To help get shoulders down farther

10. A. Proper tilt of head
    B. If head is not tipped up enough, the upper teeth will superimpose C1, C2 area; if the head is tipped too much, the base of the skull will superimpose this area.

Self-Test

My score = _____ %

Directions: Take this self-test only after completing all the review exercises and laboratory activities in this chapter. Complete directions including grading requirements are described in the front pages of this workbook and in the self-test of Chapter 1.

Test

There are 88 blanks. Each correct blank is worth 1.1 points. (Spelling is important so correct any misspellings as you grade your test.)

1. What is the major distinctive feature of all cervical vertebrae which makes them different from any other vertebrae? _transverse foramina_

2. What is the one feature of all thoracic vertebrae making them different from all other vertebrae? _____
    facets for articulation with ribs

3. The joints between the head of each rib and the bodies of the thoracic vertebrae are called? _____
    costovertebral joints

4. Fill in the correct anatomical term for the following vertebrae:

    A. C2 _axis_   C. C1 _atlas_

    B. C7 _vertebra prominens_

5. The column of bone on a typical cervical vertebra between the superior and inferior articular processes is called the _articular pillar_.

6. Matching: Match the anatomy best demonstrated on the following by placing a 1 or 2 in each blank.

    A. _1_ lateral thoracic

    B. _2_ 70° obli. thoracic

    C. _2_ lateral cervical   1. Intervertebral foramina

    D. _1_ 45° obli. cervical   2. Zygapophyseal joints

    E. _1_ lateral lumbar

    F. _2_ 45° obli. lumbar

7. Matching: Select the correct zygapophyseal joints which would be visualized on the following obliques.

    Posterior obliques: A. _2_ Thoracic / cervical _foramen_
    LPO RPO
                          B. _1_ Lumbar   1. Closest to film

    Anterior obliques: C. _1_ Thoracic / cervical   2. Farthest away from film
    RAO LAO
                          D. _2_ Lumbar

8. Which anterior oblique would demonstrate the same structures as a LPO? _____*RAO*_____

9. Fill in the correct intervertebral foramina (right or left) which would be visualized on the following <u>cervical</u> spine.

   A. LAO ____*left*____   B. RAO ____*right*____   C. RPO ____*left*____

10. Fill in the correct topographical landmark corresponding to the level of the following vertebrae:

   A. C3 ____*gonion*____   F. T4-T5 (anteriorly) *sternal angle*

   B. C1 ____*mastoid tip*____   G. T2-T3(anteriorly) *jugular notch*

   C. T7 (anteriorly) *3"-4' below jugular notch*   H. T10 (anteriorly) *xiphoid tip*

   D. C4-5 (anteriorly) *thyroid cartilage*

   E. T1 (anteriorly) (a) *1-2" above jugular notch*

      (posteriorly) (b) *vertebra prominens*

11. Fill in the correct central ray location and the direction and degrees of angle of the central ray where indicated for the following:

	CR location	Degree and direction of angle
A. Lateral thoracic	(a) *T7*	
B. AP cervical	(a) *C4-C5*	(b) *15°-20° cephalic*
C. Posterior obli. cervical	(a) *C4*	(b) *15° cephalic*
D. AP thoracic	(a) *T7*	
E. Anterior obli. cervical	(a) *C4*	(b) *15°-20° caudal*

12. To demonstrate the right zygapophyseal joints on the thoracic spine would require a __*L*__ PO (R or L) or a __*R*__ AO (R or L) rotated __*20*__ degrees from a lateral or __*70*__ degrees from an AP or PA.

13. What position would best demonstrate the <u>intervertebral foramina</u> on the following?

   A. Lumbar spine ____*lateral*____

   B. Cervical spine ____*45° oblique*____

   C. Thoracic spine ____*lateral*____

14. The "breathing technique" is commonly used for the (a) ____*lateral*____ position of the (b) ____*thoracic*____ spine.

15. What is the name of the position commonly used to demonstrate the following?

   A. Cervicothoracic region *C4-T3* ____*swimmers, twining*____

   B. C1 and C2, odontoid area ____*open mouth*____

16. What can be done to help get the shoulders down on an erect lateral cervical spine?

exhale + push down
sandbags

17. If the lateral and oblique cervical spine projections are taken in an erect position, a __72__ inch SID is used.

18. Which specific vertebrae have one full facet on each side of the vertebra? _T11, T12_

19. Which of the joints between the ribs and spine are present only on T1 through T10 vertebrae? _____

costotransverse

20. Label the following anatomical parts and joints from these drawings of a typical thoracic vertebra.

A. _pedicle_

B. _body_

C. _intervertebral foramen_

D. _spinous process_

E. _inferior articular process_

F. _transverse process_

G. _superior articular process_

Posterior　　　　　　　　　　　　　Anterior

Lateral View　　　　　Fig. 9-6

H. _spinous process_

I. _costotransverse_ joint

J. _rib_

K. _costovertebral_ joint

L. _body_

M. _facet for head of rib_

N. _pedicle_

O. _facet for tubercle of rib_

P. _transverse process_

Q. _lamina_

Posterior

Anterior

Superior View　　　　　Fig. 9-7

21. Label the following superior view drawing of a typical cervical vertebra.

A. transverse process

B. pedicle

C. lamina

D. bifid tip of spinous process

E. spinous process

F. transverse foramen

G. body

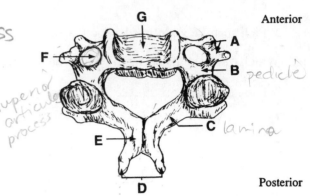

Superior View   Fig. 9-8

22. Label the following two drawings of C1 and C2.

A. dens (odontoid)

B. superior articular process

C. transverse foramen

D. inferior articular process

E. spinous process

F. lamina

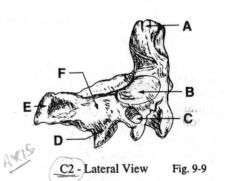

C2 - Lateral View   Fig. 9-9

G. anterior arch

H. transverse process

I. transverse foramen

J. posterior arch

K. superior articular process

L. lateral mass

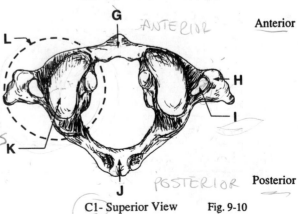

C1- Superior View   Fig. 9-10

Answers to Self-Test

1. Presence of transverse foramina

2. Presence of facets for articulation with ribs

3. Costovertebral joints

4. A. Axis
   B. Vertebra prominens
   C. Atlas

5. articular pillar

6. A. 1
   B. 2
   C. 2
   D. 1
   E. 1
   F. 2

7. A. 2
   B. 1
   C. 1
   D. 2

8. Right (RAO)

9. A. Left
   B. Right
   C. Left

10. A. Gonion
    B. Mastoid tip
    C. 3-4" below jugular notch
    D. Thyroid cartilage
    E. (a) 1-2 inches above jugular notch
       (b) Vertebra prominens
    F. Sternal angle
    G. Jugular notch
    H. Xiphoid tip

11. A. (a) T7
    B. (a) Enter at C4-5 (b) 15-20° cephalad
    C. (a) C4 (b) 15° cephalad
    D. (a) T7
    E. (a) C4 (b) 15-20° caudal

12. L, R, 20, 70

13. A. Lateral
    B. 45° oblique
    C. Lateral

14. (a) lateral (b) thoracic

15. A. Swimmer's position
    B. Open mouth AP

16. Take exposure on exhalation and relax shoulders, holding weights to pull down shoulders if necessary.

17. 72

18. T11 & 12

19. Costotransverse joints

20. A. Pedicle
    B. Body
    C. Intervertebral foramen
    D. Spinous process
    E. Inferior articular process
    F. Transverse process
    G. Superior articular process

    H. Spinous process
    I. Costotransverse
    J. Rib
    K. Costovertebral
    L. Body
    M. Facet for head of rib
    N. Pedicle
    O. Facet for tubercle of rib
    P. Transverse process
    Q. Lamina

21. A. Transverse process
    B. Pedicle
    C. Lamina
    D. Bifid tip of spinous process
    E. Spinous process
    F. Transverse foramen
    G. Body

22. A. Dens (odontoid process)
    B. Superior articular process
    C. Transverse foramen
    D. Inferior articular process
    E. Spinous process
    F. Lamina

    G. Anterior arch
    H. Transverse process
    I. Transverse foramen
    J. Posterior arch
    K. Superior articular process
    L. Lateral mass

Chapter 10
Bony Thorax
(Sternum and Ribs)

Rationale

You have already discovered that it is not enough just to place a patient in a certain position or follow blindly a certain set routine to produce quality radiographs. A thorough and accurate knowledge of normal anatomy as well as understanding of variations related to the type of injury or disease to be investigated, separate the robot-like button pusher from the professional radiologic technologist. You must understand why certain positions or projections for the ribs and sternum are superior to any others depending on the area of interest and the part to be radiographed.

The red bone marrow of the ribs and sternum are important sites of erythrocyte and granular leukocyte formation and, as such, are very sensitive to radiation damage. Your level of competence should be such so as to minimize or eliminate entirely any extra exposure related to unnecessary radiographs or additional exposures due to repeats. Good radiographs of the ribs and/or sternum will be a definite challenge to you as a radiographer.

Chapter Objectives

After you have completed **all** the activities of this chapter you will be able, with at least 80% accuracy, to: (applicable to a written and/or oral examination and demonstration)

___ 1. Identify, on both drawings and radiographs, all anatomy of the sternum and ribs as described in this chapter of the textbook and/or audio-visuals.

___ 2. Identify any pair of ribs as true, false, or floating ribs.

___ 3. Identify on radiographs, the anterior and posterior ends of any rib.

___ 4. Classify all joints in the bony thorax as to **structural classification, mobility classification** and **movement type**.

___ 5. List the basic projections, type and size of film holder, central ray location, and anatomy best demonstrated for radiographic positioning of the sternum and ribs.

___ 6. Simulate on a model and/or phantom the basic projections of the sternum and ribs.

___ 7. List the variations in breathing instructions, SID, exposure length, and kVp which can be used to advantage when radiographing the sternum in the RAO position.

___ 8. Identify all visible anatomical structures of the bony thorax as described in the textbook and/or audio-visuals.

___ 9. Critique each radiograph based on evaluation criteria provided in the textbook and/or audio-visuals.

___ 10. Discriminate between those radiographs which are acceptable and those which are unacceptable because of exposure factors, collimation or positioning errors.

___ 11. Given the necessary equipment and a simulated patient (articulated phantom or sectional phantom), produce diagnostic radiographs for the basic projections of the sternum and ribs.

Prerequisite

The prerequisite knowledge requirement for this chapter is an understanding of radiographic terminology and the principles of exposure, radiation protection, and positioning as described in Chapter 1. Chapter 2 on the chest also contains much information on both anatomy and positioning which aids in understanding the anatomy and positioning of the bony thorax. It is strongly advised that successful completion of both Chapters 1 and 2 be made mandatory prerequisites for this chapter.

Recommended Supplementary References

The following supplementary references, which are described in more detail in Chapter 1, are listed in a suggested order of importance and value to understanding this material.

1. *Merrill's ...*, Vol 1, pp 364-393

2. *Clark's ...*, pp 182-190

3. *Eisenberg ...*, pp 149-161

Learning Exercises

The following review exercises should be completed only after careful study of the associated pages in the textbook and/or audio-visuals as indicated by each exercise.

After completing each of these individual exercises, check your answers with the answer sheets which follow before continuing to the next exercise.

Part I. RADIOGRAPHIC ANATOMY

Review Exercise A   Anatomy of the Ribs and Sternum   Textbook: pp 297-301
Audio-visuals: Unit 15, slides 1-18

1. The bony thorax consists of the (a)_*clavicle*_ anteriorly, the (b) _*scapula*_ *thoracic vertebrae*

    posteriorly, and the (c) _*12*_ pairs of (d) _*ribs*_ in between.

2. Name the superior or upper division of the sternum:
    *manubrium*

3. What three names refer to the central or middle portion of the sternum?

    A. _*body*_

    B. _*corpus*_

    C. _*gladiolus*_

4. A. What name refers to the most inferior or distal part of the sternum? *xiphoid process*

    B. This part consists of cartilage during infancy and youth and doesn't become totally ossified until about

    age _*25 40*_.

5. A. What is the average length of the central or longest part of the sternum? _*4" (10 cm)*_

    B. The union of the four parts of this section of the sternum begins at (a) _*puberty*_ and is not

    completed until about age (b)_*40 25*_.

6. What is the name which applies to the junction of the manubrium and the body of the sternum?   (This is

    used as a positioning landmark.) _*sternal angle*_

7. Identify the vertebrae which are at the level of the following parts of the sternum:
    (These can be used as palpable landmarks to locate specific vertebrae.)

    A. Jugular notch _*T2 -T3*_

    B. Sternal angle _*T4 -T5*_

    C. Xiphoid process _*T 10*_

8. What is the preferred name of the superior border of the manubrium? Also list the two additional names which can be used for this important landmark.

    A. (Preferred) _jugular notch_

    B. _suprasternal notch_

    C. _manubrial notch_

9. What is the tissue or substance which connects the first seven pairs of ribs directly to the sternum?

    costocartilage

10. The anterior end of which rib connects to the sternum at the level of the sternal angle? _1st → sternal notch 1st 2nd_

11. How many pairs of ribs connect directly to the sternum by way of their own individual costocartilage?

    _7_

12. Do the last two pairs of ribs connect to the sternum by way of costocartilage? _no_

13. What term applies to the most inferior five pairs of ribs? _false ribs_

14. A. Which ribs are considered true ribs? _1-7_

    B. Why are these termed _true ribs_ as opposed to false ribs? _they're directly attached to the sternum_

15. A. The _final two_ pairs of ribs, in addition to being false ribs, are also termed _floating ribs_.

    B. Why are they called this? _they're not attached to the sternum_ _they're not connected anteriorly at all_

16. The 8th, 9th, and 10th pairs of ribs possess costocartilage. To what structure does this costocartilage attach? _the 7th rib (costocartilage)_

17. The head, neck, and tubercle of a typical rib would be located near the _vertebral_ (sternal or vertebral) end of the rib.

18. In the anatomic position, the _sternal_ (sternal or vertebral) end of each rib is more inferior.

19. What term describes the part of the rib between the vertebral and sternal ends? _angle_ _shaft or body_

20. Which three structures lie within the costal groove at the lower inside margin of each rib? (making an injury to these parts of the ribs very painful)

    A. arteries

    B. veins

    C. nerves

21. Which pair of ribs is the most sharply curved and the most vertical? 1st

22. Which pair of ribs is the longest? 8th 7th

23. The thorax is the widest at the lateral margin of either the 8th or the 9th pair of ribs.

24. Name the parts of the sternum and ribs as labeled on this drawing. (Give the preferred name.)

    A. 2nd rib

    B. clavicle

    C. Sternoclavicular joint

    D. jugular notch

    E. facet for 1st costocartilage

    F. Sternal angle

    G. body   corpus gladiolus

    H. xiphoid process

    I. 3rd rib costocartilage

    J. 7th rib costocartilage

    K. 10th rib costocartilage

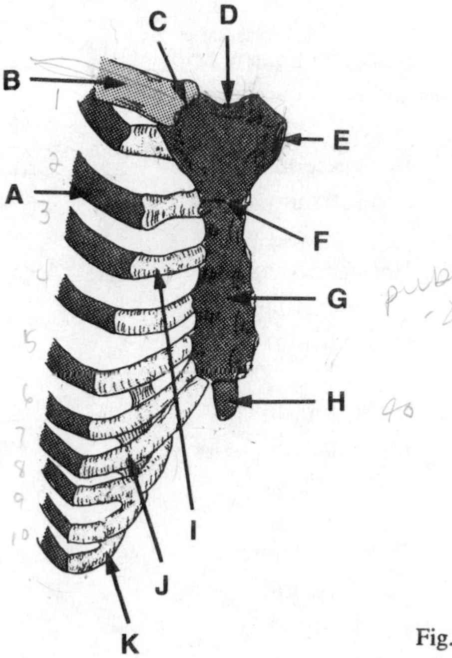

Fig. 10-1

25. Name the labeled parts of a typical rib on this drawing.

    A. angle

    B. vertebral or posterior end

    C. head

    D. neck

    E. tubercle

    F. shaft

    G. sternal or anterior end

    H. costal groove

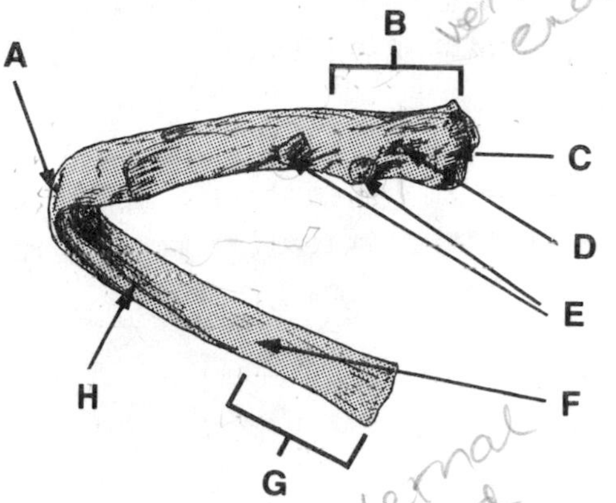

Fig. 10-2

26. What is the name of the only bony joint which connects the upper limb to the bony thorax?

S-C joint   _sternoclavicular_

27. Fill in the following blanks pertaining to the joints of the bony thorax.

A. Fibrous	D. Synarthrodial	*-no movement*	
B. Cartilaginous	E. Amphiarthrodial	*-some mov*	
C. Synovial	F. Diarthrodial	*-free moveme*	

Name of Joint		Structural Classification (A, B, or C)	Mobility Classification (D, E, or F)	Movement Type (if any)
A. Between anterior rib and costocartilage	_costochondral_	_B_	_D_	_none_
B. Between clavicle and sternum	_sternoclavicular_	_C_	_F_	_gliding_
C. Between 1st rib (costocartilage) and sternum	_sternocostal_	_B_	_D_	_none_
D. Between 5th rib (costocartilage) and sternum	_sternocostal_	_C_	_F_	_gliding_
E. Between thoracic vertebra and head of rib	_costovertebral_	_C_	_F_	_gliding_
F. Between thoracic vertebra and tubercle of rib	_costotransverse_	_C_	_F_	_gliding_

techniques

15 at 70 w/ grid
5 at 70 w/o grid
(divide mas by 3)
15 at 70 w/ detail screen,
no grid
(no change)

Part II. RADIOGRAPHIC POSITIONING

Review Exercise B   Positioning of Sternum and Ribs   Textbook: pp 302-311
Audio-visuals: Unit 15, slides 19-36

1. For the following, list the basic projections and/or positions, size and placement of cassette, and centering point.

		Basic Projections and/or Positions	Size & Placement of Cassette	Centering Point
A.	Sternum	1(a) RAO	(b) 10×12 LW	(c) mid-sternum
		2(a) lateral	(b) 10×12 LW	(c) mid-sternum
B.	Ribs, injury to right posterior rib cage (Below diaphragm)	1(a) ~~AP~~ PA	(b) 14×17 LW or CW	(c) T7
		2(a) RPO	(b) 14×17 CW	(c) midway btw xiphoid tip & lower ribcage
C.	Ribs, injury to left anterior axillary ribs (Above diaphragm)	1(a) PA	(b) 14×17 LW or CW	(c) T7
		2(a) ~~LAO~~ RAO	(b) 14×17 LW	(c) T7

2. When radiographing the sternum, why is an RAO preferable to the LAO?

so the sternum is superimposed over the heart shadow

3. Why is a slight RAO position better than a straight PA when radiographing the sternum?

to throw the sternum away from the thoracic spine

4. How much does the body need to be obliqued for the RAO sternum?

A. On a large deep-chested patient? 15°

B. On a small thin-chested patient? 20° ✓

5. Under ideal conditions, select the better of each pair of technical factors which would produce the best quality radiograph of an RAO sternum by placing a check in the correct blank.

A. (a) ✗ 30-40 inch SID   or   (b)_____44-46 inch SID

B. (a) ✗ shallow breathing   or   (b)_____ suspended inspiration

C. (a) ✗ 3-4 second exposure   or   (b)_____ .5 to 1 second exposure

D. (a)_____ 90-92 kVp   or   (b) ✗ 60-70 kVp

6. Explain your selection of SID in part 5A above.

shorter SID will magnify + blur structures farther from the film   and greater magnification and blur overlying ribs

7. Support your selection of breathing instructions in part 5B above.

breathing technique to blur out lung markings + ribs

8. Support your selection of exposure time in part 5C above.

long exposure time with breathing technique

_8 ft._

9. Support your selection of kVp in part 5D above.

low kV so sternum isn't over-penetrated

10. Which three positions can be used to obtain a lateral sternum.

A. _erect lateral_

B. _recumbent lateral_

C. _lateral decubitus_

11. Which part of the sternum is easiest to palpate when positioning for a sternum?

jugular notch

12. Where should the arms be placed when positioning for an erect lateral sternum?

behind back

13. Can a satisfactory lateral sternum be produced using a <u>high kVp</u> lateral chest technique?

no - high kVp will over-penetrate

14. What term describes bleeding into the thoracic cavity?

hemothorax

15. What term describes the accumulation of air in the pleural space? _pneumothorax_

16. Which requires the greater exposure factors, ribs which are above or below the level of the diaphragm?

below

17. Which anterior landmark can be used to determine if a rib injury is above or below the diaphragm?

xiphoid tip (at T-10)

18. Above the diaphragm ribs would be exposed on _inspiration_ (inspiration or expiration).

19. Below the diaphragm ribs would be exposed on _expiration_ (inspiration or expiration).

20. The oblique position in a rib series is done primarily to show which part of the rib cage?

mid-lateral or axillary

21. Indicate which oblique(s) would be taken with rib injuries to the following areas of the rib cage: Also state if the above diaphragm (AD) or below diaphragm (BD) technique would be used.

	Oblique	AD or BD
A. Right posterior 5th rib	RPO	AD
B. Left anterior 5th rib	~~LAO~~ RAO	AD
C. Left posterior 10th rib	LPO	BD

22. The primary objective when radiographing ribs in the oblique position is to rotate the spine

away (towards or away) from the area of injury.

23. Why must the cassette be turned cross-wise when radiographing below-the-diaphragm ribs in the AP

projection? _width of the rib cage greatest at 8th or 9th ribs_

Review Exercise C   Textbook: pp 306-311

This part of the learning activity exercises needs to be carried out in a radiographic laboratory or a general diagnostic room in a radiology department. Part B can be carried out in a classroom or any room where illuminators are available.

A. Positioning Exercise

For this section you need another person or an articulated phantom to act as your patient. Practice the following until you can do each of them accurately and without hesitation. It is important to achieve both accuracy and speed in radiographic positioning. Place a check by each when you have achieved this.

Include the following details as you simulate the basic projections for each exam listed below:

- correct size and type of film holder
- correct location of central ray and correct centering of part to film
- correct placement of markers
- accurate collimation
- proper use of immobilizing devices when needed
- approximate correct exposure factors
- correct instructions to your patient as you simulate the exposure
- use of gonadal shields

___ 1. RAO sternum

___ 2. Lateral sternum (patient erect)

___ 3. Lateral sternum (patient recumbent)

___ 4. Lateral sternum (patient dorsal recumbent)

___ 5. AP ribs (above diaphragm)

___ 6. AP ribs (below diaphragm)

___ 7. Posterior oblique ribs

___ 8. Anterior oblique ribs

Optional

Using either a sectional or fully articulated phantom, produce a diagnostic radiograph for each basic projection or position of the following:

___ 1. Sternum

___ 2. Ribs (posterior and above diaphragm injury)

___ 3. Ribs (anterior and above diaphragm injury)

___ 4. Ribs (posterior and below diaphragm injury)

B. Review of Anatomy on Radiographs

Use those radiographs provided by your instructor. (These should include acceptable quality radiographs of the sternum and ribs.)

___ 1. Examine radiographs of the sternum and ribs, and identify those anatomical parts described in the textbook and/or audio-visuals.

C. Film Critique and Evaluation

Your instructor will provide various radiographs of the sternum and ribs for these exercises. Some will be optimal quality radiographs meeting all or most of the evaluation criteria described for each projection in the textbook and/or audio-visuals. Others will be less than optimal quality and several will be unacceptable, requiring a repeat exam. You should evaluate each radiograph as specified below.

Place a check by each of the following when it is completed.

___ 1. Critique each radiograph based on evaluation criteria provided for each projection in the textbook and/or audio-visuals. The following criteria guidelines can be used and checked as each radiograph is evaluated. (Additional checks can be placed to the left for each criteria guideline if more than four radiographs are evaluated.)

```
     Radiographs              Criteria Guidelines
    1  2  3  4
   __ __ __ __    a. Correct film size and correct orientation of part to film?

   __ __ __ __    b. Correct alignment and/or centering of part to film or portion of film being used?

   __ __ __ __    c. Correct collimation and CR location?

   __ __ __ __    d. Pertinent anatomy well visualized?

   __ __ __ __    e. Motion?

   __ __ __ __    f. Optimum exposure; density and/or contrast?

   __ __ __ __    g. Patient ID information and markers?

   __ __ __ __    h. Gonadal shielding correctly placed if used?
```

___ 2. Based on acceptable variances to criteria factors, determine which of these radiographs are acceptable and which are unacceptable and should have been repeated.

IMPORTANT: It is important that you have successfully carried out all of the exercises described above before taking the self-test and before going to your instructor for the chapter evaluation exam. If you neglect these exercises, you will not be able to meet all objectives for this chapter and may not receive a passing grade for this course.

Answers to Review Exercise A

1. (a) Sternum   (b) Thoracic vertebrae   (c) 12
   (d) Ribs

2. Manubrium

3. A. Body
   B. Corpus
   C. Gladiolus

4. A. Xiphoid process
   B. 40

5. A. 4 inches or 10 cm
   B. (a) Puberty   (b) 25

6. Sternal angle

7. A. T2-3
   B. T4-5
   C. T10

8. A. Jugular notch
   B. Suprasternal notch
   C. Manubrial notch

9. Costocartilage

10. 2nd rib

11. Seven

12. No

13. False ribs

14. A. 1st seven pairs
    B. Because they attach directly to sternum

15. A. Floating ribs
    B. Because they are not connected
       anteriorly

16. The costocartilage of the seventh rib

17. Vertebral

18. Sternal

19. Shaft or body

20. A. Artery
    B. Vein
    C. Nerve

21. 1st

22. 7th

23. 8th, 9th

24. A. 2nd rib
    B. Clavicle
    C. Sternoclavicular joint
    D. Jugular notch
    E. Facet for 1st costocartilage
    F. Sternal angle
    G. Body
    H. Xiphoid process
    I. Costocartilage, 3rd rib
    J. Costocartilage, 7th rib
    K. Costocartilage, 10th rib

25. A. Angle
    B. Vertebral, posterior
    C. Head
    D. Neck
    E. Tubercle
    F. Shaft
    G. Sternal, anterior
    H. Costal groove

26. Sternoclavicular joint

27. A. Costochondral, B, D, none
    B. Sternoclavicular, C, F, gliding
    C. Sternocostal, B, D, none
    D. Sternocostal, C, F, gliding
    E. Costovertebral, C, F, gliding
    F. Costotransverse, C, F, gliding

If you missed more than 13 blanks, you should review
this section again in the textbook and/or audio-visuals
before continuing.

Answers to Review Exercise B

1. A. 1(a) RAO (b) 10 x 12 LW
       (c) Mid-sternum

       2(a) Lateral (b) 10 x 12 LW
       (c) Mid-sternum

  B. 1(a) RPO (b) 14 x 17 CW
       (c) Midway between xiphoid tip and
          lower rib cage

       2(a) PA chest, erect (b) 14 x 17 LW
       or CW (c) T7

  C. 1(a) RAO (b) 14 x 17 LW (c) T7

       2(a) PA chest, erect (b) 14 x 17 LW
       or CW (c) T7

2. To project sternum over heart shadow which provides a homogeneous background density.

3. To prevent superimposition of the thoracic spine and sternum

4. A. 15 degrees
  B. 20 degrees

5. A. (a) x
  B. (a) x
  C. (a) x
  D. (b) x

6. To better visualize the sternum. Shorter SID will magnify and blur structures farther from the film.

7. Shallow breathing during exposure will blur overlying lung markings.

8. An exposure of 3 to 4 seconds will help to blur lung markings.

9. A lower kVp (60-70) will better maintain visibility and contrast of sternum.

10. A. Erect lateral
   B. Recumbent lateral
   C. Lateral decubitus (cross-table lateral)

11. Jugular notch

12. Drawn back as far as possible.

13. No, requires lower kVp to maintain contrast

14. Hemothorax

15. Pneumothorax

16. Below

17. Xiphoid tip (level of T-10)

18. Inspiration

19. Expiration

20. Mid-lateral or axillary portion.

21. A. RPO   AD
   B. RAO   AD
   C. LPO   BD

22. Away from

23. Width of thoracic cage greatest at level of 8th or 9th rib.

If you missed more than 10 blanks, you should review this section again in the textbook and/or audio-visuals before continuing.

Self-Test

My score = _____ %

Directions: Take this self-test only after completing all the review exercises and laboratory activities in this chapter. Complete directions including grading requirements are described in the front pages of this workbook and in the self-test of Chapter 1.

Test

There are 40 blanks. Each correct blank is worth 2.5 points. (Spelling is important so correct any misspellings as you grade your test.)

1. The sternum consists of three parts. Name the most superior part. _manubrium_

2. The most inferior part of the sternum is called the _xiphoid process_.

3. The junction of the manubrium with the body of the sternum is termed the _sternal angle_.

4. The superior border of the manubrium is termed the manubrial notch, the suprasternal notch, or the preferred _jugular notch_.

5. To which part of the sternum does the costocartilage of the first rib attach? _manubrium_

6. To which part of the sternum does the costocartilage of the fifth rib attach? _body_

7. The sternoclavicular joint, which is classed as a synovial/diarthrodial joint, permits which type of motion? _gliding_

8. How many pairs of ribs are considered true ribs? _7_

9. What name applies to the last five pairs of ribs? _false_

10. The head of the rib would be found at which end of a typical rib? _posterior (vertebral)_

11. Which end of each rib is most inferior? _anterior (sternal)_

12. Which pair(s) of ribs are considered floating ribs? _11th + 12th_

13. An artery, a vein, and a nerve are protected by what portion or structure of each rib? _costal groove_

14. Which pair of ribs is the longest? _7th_

15. A. The joint between the costocartilage of the (first) rib and the manubrium of the sternum forms which structural classification of joint? _cartilagenous_

    B. What mobility classification is this? _synorthrodial_
    no movement

16. A. When radiographing the sternum, which anterior oblique is preferable? _RAO_

    B. Why? _superimpose sternum over heart shadow_

17. Why is a long exposure time (3 to 4 sec.) advantageous when radiographing the sternum in the anterior oblique position? _blur out lung markings_

18. The complete union of the four parts of the body of the sternum occurs at approximately what age? _25_ *starts at puberty*

19. Generally complete ossification of the xiphoid process occurs at approximately what age? _40_

20. What is the centering point on the sternum for radiography of the sternum? _mid-sternum_

21. T4-5 is at the level of what palpable landmark of the sternum? _sternal angle_

22. The jugular notch is approximately at the level of _T2-T3_ vertebra.

23. The xiphoid process is approximately at the level of _T10_ vertebra.

24. What term describes any abnormal accumulation of <u>air</u> in the pleural space? _pneumothorax_

25. The centering point for an AP radiograph of the ribs below the diaphragm would be _midway between xiphoid + lower rib cage_.

26. To radiograph ribs in the oblique position, it is necessary to rotate what structure away from the area of the injury? _thoracic vertebrae_

27. Which oblique rib position best demonstrates the following:

    A. Left anterior <u>axillary</u> ribs? _LAO   RAO_

    B. Left posterior ribs? _LPO_

28. Would injury to the <u>8th</u> pair of ribs require an exposure technique for above diaphragm or below diaphragm? _above_

29. An oblique sternum should be taken at approximately what <u>kVp</u> range? _60-65 70_

30. A full inspiration on an average patient places the dome of the diaphragm at the level of the _10th_ posterior ribs.

31. Which pair of ribs are the most inferior true ribs? _7th_

32. What joint connects the upper limb to the bony thorax? _sternoclavicular_

33. What are the breathing instructions for:

    A. Oblique sternum? _shallow breaths   3 sec. breathe techn_

    B. Lateral sternum? _hold breath on inspiration_

    C. Oblique ribs with injury at 10th posterior ribs? _hold breath /expiration_

    D. Oblique ribs with injury at 4th anterior ribs? _hold breath /inspiration_

Answers to Self-Test

1. Manubrium

2. xiphoid process

3. sternal angle

4. jugular notch

5. Manubrium

6. Body

7. Gliding

8. Seven

9. False ribs

10. Vertebral or posterior

11. Sternal or anterior

12. 11th and 12th

13. Costal groove

14. 7th

15. A. Cartilaginous
    B. Synarthrodial

16. A. Right (RAO)
    B. To superimpose the sternum over the homogeneous heart shadow.

17. To allow breathing motion to blur out lung markings.

18. 25

19. 40

20. Mid-sternum (half-way between jugular notch and xiphoid process)

21. Sternal angle

22. T2-3

23. T10

24. Pneumothorax

25. midway between xiphoid and lower rib cage

26. Vertebral column

27. A. RAO
    B. LPO

28. Above

29. 60-70

30. 10th

31. 7th

32. Sternoclavicular

33. A. Continue breathing during exposure
    B. Hold on inspiration
    C. Hold on expiration
    D. Hold on inspiration

Chapter 11
Cranium
(Skull Series and Sella Turcica)

Rationale

Radiographic examinations involving the skull are usually considered among the most difficult of all examinations. The skull is a very compact structure involving many small but important bony structures surrounded or superimposed by other structures of the skull. This makes it very difficult to visualize many of these bony structures on radiographs.

The anatomy of the skull, including both the cranial and facial bones, is very detailed, especially those cranial bones making up the "floor" and lower "walls" of the cranial vault. To visualize many of these structures requires controlled use of displacement radiography. This requires either certain rather precise angulations of the central ray or specific obliques of the skull. An example of this is an axial AP projection of the skull which specifically demonstrates the occipital bone and the petrous pyramids of the temporal bone. This projection requires a very precise 30 degree caudal angle to the orbitomeatal line, a special positioning line of the head. This central ray angulation projects the facial bone mass caudally so it will not superimpose the specific structures being demonstrated on this projection. The same is true for visualizing the facial bones without superimposition by the dense petrous pyramids as will be described in Chapter 12.

Good skull radiography is a definite challenge and requires much effort and study before it can be mastered. The detailed anatomy of the skull is presented in such a way in the textbook and/or audio-visuals that it will allow you to learn the anatomical terms for all of these structures as well as relationships to other internal as well as external structures and landmarks.

These next three chapters involving the cranium and facial bones are complex and no pretense is made to the contrary. These will require extra time in studying the accompanying textbook and in carefully completing all of these review exercises including the laboratory activities described at the end of each chapter. It will take some concentrated effort on your part but the opportunity for you to master this material and become a good skull radiographer is there—if you are willing.

Chapter Objectives

After you have successfully completed **all** the activities of this unit, you will be able, with at least 80% accuracy, to: (applicable to a written and/or oral examination and demonstration)

___ 1. List and locate all surface landmarks and localizing lines described in this chapter.

___ 2. Identify the external landmarks which correspond to the level of the floor of the anterior cranium and the level of the petrous ridge.

___ 3. List the eight cranial bones and identify the four bones composing the calvarium or "skull cap" and the four making up the "floor" of the cranium.

___ 4. Describe the relative locations or positions of the eight cranial bones and identify on drawings and radiographs the various portions or parts of each cranial bone as described in this chapter.

___ 5. List and identify on drawings and radiographs the sutures of the skull including the areas of the six fontanels or "soft spots" on newborns.

___ 6. List the number and the names of specific adjoining cranial bones with which each cranial bone articulates.

___ 7. List the three terms describing the common shape classifications of the cranium and identify the approximate angles of the petrous pyramids for each classification.

___ 8. Describe the correct angle (caudal or cephalad), the degrees of angle and the line used to determine this angle on a PA Caldwell, and an axial AP projection.

___ 9. For a submentovertex projection, identify the line which should be as near parallel to the plane of the film as possible and describe the relationship of the central ray to this line.

___ 10. Position a model and/or phantom for each of the basic and optional projections as described in the textbook and/or audiovisuals. Include the three different ways for taking each projection which are: (a) on a routine radiographic table, (b) on a vertical head unit or erect table or grid film holder, (c) modifications for severely injured patients.

___ 11. Critique skull radiographs based on evaluation criteria provided in the textbook and/or audio-visuals.

___ 12. Discriminate between radiographs which are acceptable and those which are unacceptable due to exposure factors, collimation or positioning errors.

Prerequisite

The prerequisite knowledge requirement for this chapter is an understanding of radiographic terminology and the principles of exposure, radiation protection and positioning as described in Chapter 1. It is strongly suggested that a mandatory prerequisite for this chapter be the successful completion of Chapter 1.

Recommended Supplementary References

The following supplementary references, which are described in more detail in Chapter 1, are listed in a suggested order of importance and value to understanding this material.

1. *Merrill's ...*, Vol 2, pp 202-255

2. *Clark's ...*, pp 192-209

3. *Eisenberg ...*, pp 263-292

Learning Exercises

The following review exercises should be completed only after careful study of the associated pages in the textbook and/or audio-visuals as indicated by each exercise.

After completing, check your answers with the answer sheets following these review exercises.

Part I. RADIOGRAPHIC ANATOMY

Review Exercise A   Topographical Anatomy and Landmarks, Lines and Planes of the Cranium

Textbook: pp 313-317
Audio-visuals: Unit 10, slides 1-12

1. Fill in the total number of bones for:

    A. Cranium _____8_____

    B. Facial bones _____14_____

2. Describe the location of the following topographical landmarks of the cranium:

    A. Glabella _triangular area btw. eyebrows + above ridge of nose_

    B. Acanthion _where nose + upper lip meet_

    C. Mental point _midpoint of the chin_

    D. Superciliary ridge (arch) _arch of bone above each eye_

    E. Supraorbital groove _groove above the eyebrow_

    F. Nasion _depression at bridge of the nose_

    G. Angle (gonion) _lower posterior angle on side of jaw_

    H. Vertex _top of the cranium_

    I. Inion _bump on back of head_

3. Which of the above landmarks corresponds to the level of the floor of the anterior fossa of the cranium?

    supraorbital groove (SOG)

4. Fill in the correct term describing the following five landmarks relating to the eye or rim of orbit:

    A. Medial junction of two eyelids _inner canthus_

    B. Lateral junction of the two eyelids _outer canthus_

    C. Superior rim of orbit _supraorbital margin (SOM)_

    D. Inferior rim of orbit _infraorbital margin (IOM)_

    E. Lateral aspect of orbital rim _mid-lateral orbital margin_

5. Fill in the correct term or a second term for the following landmarks.

    A. EAM _external auditory meatus_

    B. TEA _top of the ear attachment_

    C. SOM _supraorbital margin_

    D. IOM _infraorbital margin_

6. The orbit is (a)_conical_ in shape and extends (b)_posteriorly_ (anteriorly or posteriorly) from the base.   _base is front of eye_

7. The circular rim of the orbit which can be palpated is actually the _base_ of the orbit.

8. What is the external landmark corresponding to the petrous ridge? _top of ear attachment (TEA)_

9. Fill in the correct term describing the following planes and lines:

    A. Divides the body into right and left halves   _midsagittal_

    B. Describes the imaginary line drawn between the pupils of the eyes.   _interpupillary_

    C. The line connecting the glabella to the EAM   _glabellomeatal_

    D. The line connecting the outer canthus of the eye to the EAM.   GML   _orbitomeatal_ (radiographic) baseline

    E. Describes the line between the infraorbital margin and the EAM.   IOML   _infraorbitalmeatal_ (Reids)

    F. The line between the acanthion and the EAM.   _acanthiomeatal_

    G. The line between the "chin" and the EAM.   _mentomeatal_

    H. The line between the glabella and the anterior aspect of the alveolar process of the maxilla.   _glabelloalveolar_

10. Reid's base line, or just *base line* is also used occasionally to describe the _infraorbital-meatal line_.

11. Which line should be perpendicular to the film on a true lateral skull? _orbitomeatal interpupillary line_

12. Which body plane of the head must be parallel to the plane of the film on a true lateral skull? _midsagittal_

Review Exercise B   Anatomy of Cranium

Textbook: pp 317-323
Audio-visuals: Unit 10, slides 13-34

1. What is the correct anatomical term describing the skull cap? (a)___calvarium___

   What are the names of the four bones making up this portion of the skull? (b)___frontal___

   right and left (c)___parietal___ and (d)___occipital___.

2. What are the names of the additional four cranial bones which primarily make up the floor of the cranium?

   The right and left (a)___temporal___, the (b)___sphenoid___, and the (c)___ethmoid___.

3. The frontal bone can be divided into two portions, the vertical or (a)___squamous___ portion and

   the horizontal or (b)___orbital___ portion.

4. The ridge of bone under each eyebrow is called the ___superciliary ridge___ arch

5. The portion of the frontal bone forming the superior aspect of each orbit is the ___orbital plate___

6. Two bones which primarily make up the walls of the calvarium or skull cap are the right and left

   ___parietal bones___.

7. The widest portion of the skull is found between the ___parietal tubercles___ of the two bones
   described in question number 6.

8. Answer the following questions on the joints or articulations of the skull (excluding the temporomandibular joint, TMJ):

   A. The correct anatomical term for these joints? ___sutures___

   B. Structural classification of these joints? ___fibrous___

   C. Functional or mobility classification of these joints? ___synarthrodial___

   D. Are these movable or immovable joints? ___immovable___

   E. Separates the frontal from the two parietals. ___coronal suture___

   F. Separates the two parietals. ___sagittal___

   G. Separates the two parietals from the occipital bone. ___lambdoidal___

   H. Separates the parietals from the temporals. ___squamosal___

   I. The anterior end of the sagittal suture is called the ___bregma___   ANTERIOR FONTANEL

   J. The posterior end of the sagittal suture is called the ___lambda___   POSTERIOR FONTANEL

   K. The areas described in Parts I and J are "soft spots" in newborns and are called the anterior and

   posterior ___fontanels___.

(continued on next page)

8. *(continued)*

L. The "soft spots" located at the sphenoid angle of the parietal bone on each side of the head are called (a) *sphenoid fontanels* , on an adult this point (which can be used for specific cranial measurements) is called the (b) *pterion* .

M. The second lateral "soft spot" located at the mastoid angle of the parietal bone on each side is called the (a) *mastoid fontanel* , and on an adult is called the (b) *asterion* .

N. Which of the six "soft spots" of the cranium is the largest and doesn't close until about 18 months of age? *anterior fontanel* (bregma)

O. What are the small irregular bones called which sometimes develop in adults at the "soft spots?" *sutural or Wormian bones*

9. The posterior and somewhat inferior portion of the calvarium is formed by the single *occipital* bone.

10. The large hole or opening in the bone described in question 9 is called the *foramen magnum*.

11. The two oval convex articular surfaces on each side of this large opening at the base of the skull are called (a) *occipital condyles* or (b) *lateral condylar portions*

12. The articulation between the skull and cervical spine is called the *occipito- atalantal* joint..

    ATLAS

13. Identify the labeled parts of the following drawings:

    A. *coronal suture*
    B. *bregma (anterior fontanel)*
    C. *squamosal suture*
    D. *lambda (posterior fontanel)*
    E. *lambdoidal suture*
    F. *inion*
    G. *asterion (mastoid fontanel)*
    H. *pterion (sphenoid fontanel)*

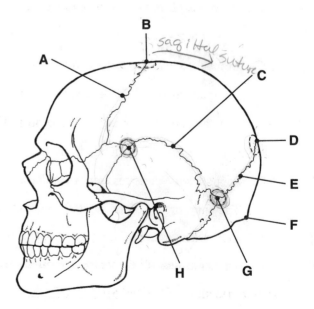

sagittal suture

Fig. 11-1

222

13. *(continued)*

I. frontal eminence

J. supraorbital groove

K. superciliary arch

L. orbital plate of frontal bone

M. nasion

N. glabella

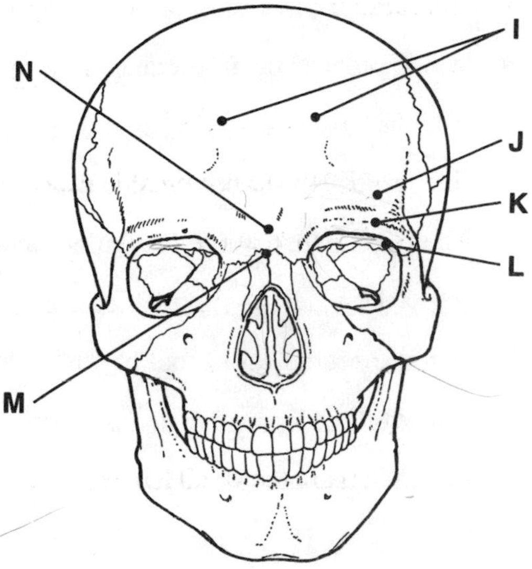

Fig. 11-2

14. The two lateral condylar processes *(occipital condyles)* are part of the ___occipital___ bone. (Hint: these processes help make up a joint involving the skull.)

15. The ___temporal___ bones house the organs of hearing and balance.

16. The ___sphenoid___ bone is the primary anchor bone for all eight cranial bones.

17. The ___ethmoid___ bone lies primarily below the floor of the cranium.

18. The thin "wall" portion of the temporals is called the ___squamous___ portion *squamous, mastoid, petrous* (similar to name of the suture at upper border of temporal).

19. The temporal bone contains a process of bone called the (a)___zygomatic___ process, which meets another process of a facial bone to make up a prominent arch of bone called the (b)___zygomatic arch___.

20. The temporal bone contains a fossa called the ___temporomandibular___ fossa which helps form the only diarthrodial or freely movable joint of the skull.

21. A slender process of the temporal bone projecting downward is called the ___styloid___ process.

22. The thick portion of the temporal bone directly posterior to the EAM which contains air cells is called the (a)___mastoid___ portion, which has a small, somewhat "blunt" process or tip projecting downward called the (b)___mastoid tip (process)___.

23. The petrous portions of the temporal bones are the thickest and most dense bones in the skull and are sometimes also called the (a)___petrous pyramids___ or ___pars petrosa___. The upper edges of these portions are often called the (b)___petrous ridges___.

24. The central depression of the sphenoid which looks like a saddle is called the (a) _sella turcica_ which protects the important (b) _pituitary_ (hypophysis) gland.

25. The back of this "saddle" is called the (a) _dorsum sellae_, which contains two small ear-like projections of bone called the (b) _posterior clinoid processes_

26. The two small, ear-like projections anterior to the "saddle" are called the (a) _anterior clinoid processes_, which are attached to a pair of triangular shaped and nearly horizontal projections of the sphenoid called the (b) _lesser wings_.

27. The shallow depression just posterior to the dorsum sellae which forms a continuous groove to the foramen magnum and provides a base of support for the pons portion of the brain is called the _clivus_.

28. The sphenoid bone contains four processes projecting downward:

   A.   The two more lateral and somewhat flat processes are called _lateral pterygoid proce_

   B.   The two medial and more pointed processes are called the _medial pterygoid proces_

   C.   The two hook-like projections extending from the medial processes are called the _pterygoid hamu_

29. The three pairs of small openings (for nerves and blood vessels) in the greater wing of the sphenoid are the (a) _foramen rotundum_, (b) _foramen ovale_ and (c) _foramen spinosum_.

30. The sphenoid articulates with _all seven_ other cranial bones.

31. Answer the following questions regarding the ethmoid bone.

   A.   The small horizontal portion located in the ethmoid notch of the frontal bone is the _cribiform plate_.

   B.   The superior projection which has an appearance of a rooster's comb is the _crista galli_.

   C.   The portion projecting downward in the midline to help form the bony nasal septum is the _perpendicular plate_.

   D.   The two lateral masses, also called the lateral _labyrinths_, contain air cells and are suspended inferiorly from the under-surface of the horizontal portion of the ethmoid.

   E.   Extending medially and downward from these lateral masses are thin, scroll-like projections called the superior and middle (a) _nasal conchae_, sometimes called (b) _turbinates_.

   F.   The ethmoid articulates with two cranial bones, the (a) _frontal_ and (b) _sphenoid_.

32. Fill in the following from the labeled drawings:

Temporal & Sphenoid Bones

A. zygomatic process

B. left greater wing of sphenoid bone

C. squamous portion of temporal bone

D. mastoid process

E. EAM

F. styloid process

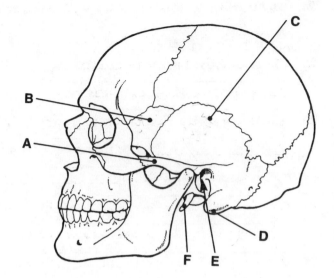

Fig. 11-3

Sphenoid Bone

G. anterior clinoid process

H. posterior clinoid process

I. dorsum sellae

J. clivus

K. sella turcica

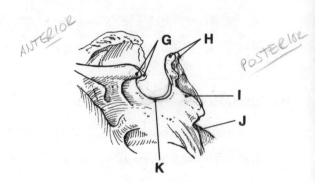

Fig. 11-4

Ethmoid and Sphenoid Bone

L. perpendicular plate of ethmoid

M. crista galli of ethmoid

N. cribiform plate of ethmoid

O. pterygoid process of sphenoid

P. pterygoid hamulus of sphenoid

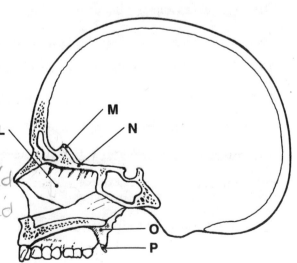

Midsagittal Section   Fig. 11-5

32. (continued)

Ethmoid, Sphenoid, Occipital and Frontal Bones

Q. crista galli of ethmoid

R. cribiform plate of ethmoid

S. lesser wing of sphenoid

T. greater wing of sphenoid

U. foramen ovale of sphenoid

V. foramen spinosum of sphenoid

W. petrous pyramid of temporal bone

X. foramen magnum of occipital bone

Y. posterior clinoid process of sphenoid

Z. sella turcica of sphenoid

a. anterior clinoid processes

b. orbital plate of frontal bone

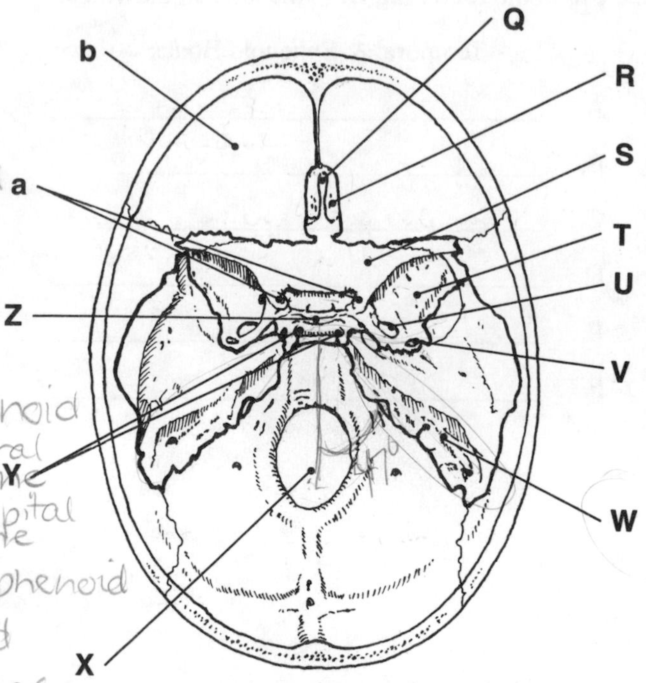

Superior View
(Top of Skull Removed)

Fig. 11-6

33. The frontal bone articulates with four cranial bones, the right and left (a) parietals , the
(b) sphenoid and the (c) ethmoid .

34. The parietal articulates with five cranial bones: (a) frontal , (b) occipital
(c) temporal , (d) sphenoid , and (e) parietal (other)

35. The occipital articulates with six bones: right and left (a) parietals , right and left
(b) temporals , the (c) sphenoid , and the (d) atlas (C1)

36. A lateral measurement of the cranium should be made in the area of the largest diameter which is between
the two (a) parietal eminences, which averages (b) 15 centimeters.

37. The anteroposterior measurement should be made between the (a) frontal eminence and the
(b) external occipital protuberance , which averages (c) 19 centimeters.

38. Fill in the correct shape classifications and the approximate angle between the petrous pyramids and the
midsagittal plane for the following:

A. Average shaped head   mesocephalic ,   47 degrees

B. Short broad head   brachycephalic ,   ±54 degrees

C. Long narrow head   dolichocephalic ,   ±40 degrees

Part II. RADIOGRAPHIC POSITIONING

Review Exercise C   Positioning of the Cranium and Sella Turcica

Textbook: pp 324-339
Audio-visuals: Unit 15, slides 19-36

1. List the three basic and the one optional projection most commonly included in a skull series. List second terms where more than one term is commonly used.

   Basic: A. _AP axial (Townes)_

              B. _lateral_

              C. _PA 0° or PA 15° Caldwell_

   Optional: D. _submentovertex (basilar)_

2. When positioning for a lateral skull projection, which line should be placed perpendicular to the side of the table? _infraorbitomeatal (IOML) interpupillary_

3. Indicate which way the 10 x 12 cassette should be placed (crosswise or lengthwise) on the following projections taken on a radiographic table.

   A.   Lateral   _crosswise_

   B.   PA or Caldwell   _lengthwise_

   C.   AP axial   _lengthwise_

   D.   Submentovertex   _lengthwise_

4. What are the two lines or planes which should be checked carefully to insure a true lateral skull position? Indicate if these should be parallel or perpendicular to the plane of the film.

   A. _midsagittal plane_   _parallel_

   B. _interpupillary_   _perpendicular_

5. Describe the central ray location for the following two methods commonly used in centering for a lateral skull projection.

   A.   Center entire cranium to film: _2" superior to EAM_

   B.   Center sella turcica to film: _3/4" anterior & 3/4" superior to EAM_

6. There is a _7+8_ degree difference between the OML and IOML.

7. In checking a lateral skull radiograph for possible rotation or tilt, what four pairs of anatomical structures should be directly superimposed?

   A. _mandibular rami_   C. _wings of sphenoid_

   B. _orbital roofs_   D. _external auditory canals_

8. Fill in the correct lines and/or planes which should be perpendicular to the film on the following positions or projections:

   A. Lateral: _interpupillary_ line

   B. PA Caldwell: (a)_orbitomeatal_ line and (b)_midsagittal_ plane

   C. AP axial: (a)_orbitomeatal_ line and (b)_midsagittal_ plane
      Townes

9. Fill in the correct angle, number of degrees and the correct line used to determine this angle on the following:

		Caudal or Cephalad	Degrees of Angle		Line
A.	PA Caldwell	(a) _caudal_	(b) _15°_	(c)	_OML_
B.	Reversal of Caldwell for severely injured	(a) _cephalic_	(b) _15°_	(c)	_OML_
C.	AP axial Townes (AP)	(a) _caudal_	(b) _30°_	(c)	_OML_

10. For an AP axial projection, the central ray should be angled (a)_30_ degrees caudal if the orbitomeatal ~~OML~~ line is perpendicular to the film and (b)_37_ degrees if the infraorbitomeatal line is perpendicular. _IOML_

11. The dorsum sellae and posterior clinoids are projected **into the foramen magnum** on which sella turcica projection(s)? _PA , PA axial (25° cephalic) 37° AP axial_

12. The dorsum sellae and posterior clinoids are projected just **superior to the foramen magnum,** superimposing the occipital bone, with the _30° AP axial_ sella turcica projection.

13. What two intracranial structures are demonstrated in profile on a true lateral skull?

    (a)_sella turcica_ and (b)_clivus_ .

14. Complete the following for a submentovertex projection of the skull:

    A. The patient should be positioned so the_IOML_ line is parallel to the plane of the film.

    B. The central ray must be perpendicular to the _infraorbitomeatal_ line.

    C. If the correct line was perpendicular to the central ray, then the condyles of the mandible will be projected (a)_anterior_ (anterior or posterior) to the (b)_petrous pyramid_

15. The projections best demonstrating the following:

    A. Sella Turcica (a)_lateral_ and (b)_AP axial_

    B. Petrous Pyramids (ridges) (a)_AP axial_ and (b)_~~PA~~ submentovert_

16. The internal auditory canals are best demonstrated on which projection?_PA Caldwell 0°_

17. Which trauma skull projection is essential for visualizing inner cranial air/fluid levels?_crosstable lateral (horizontal beam)_

Review Exercise D   Laboratory Activity   Textbook: pp 328-339

Part A of this learning activity exercise needs to be carried out in a radiographic laboratory or a general diagnostic room in a radiology department. Parts B and D can be carried out in a classroom or any room where illuminators are available.

A. Positioning Exercise

For this section you need another person or an articulated phantom to act as your patient. Practice the following until you can do each of them accurately and without hesitation. It is important to achieve both accuracy and speed in radiographic positioning. Place a check by each when you have achieved this.

Include the following details as you simulate the basic projections for each exam listed below:

- correct size and type of film holder
- correct location and angle of central ray
- correct centering of part to film
- correct placement of markers
- accurate collimation
- proper use of immobilizing devices when needed
- approximate correct exposure factors
- correct instructions to your patient as you simulate the exposure

___ 1. Table top lateral and PA Caldwell projections.

___ 2. Table top AP axial and submentovertex projections.

___ 3. Erect (with head unit if available or with erect table or other erect grid-film holder), lateral, PA Caldwell, AP axial and submentovertex projections.

___ 4. Severely injured patient who cannot be moved from a supine position on a stretcher. (Spinal injury has been ruled out by a cross-table lateral cervical spine). Take a cross-table lateral projection, AP projection to replace routine PA Caldwell and AP axial (Towne) projection.

___ 5. Special projections for sella turcica (erect or table top).

Optional: Using either a sectional or a full articulated phantom, produce a diagnostic radiograph for the following:

___ 1. Cross-table lateral projection.

___ 2. AP Axial (Towne) and modified AP to replace PA Caldwell on severely injured patient.

___ 3. Table top lateral and PA Caldwell projections.

___ 4. Submentovertex projection (disarticulated skull phantom only).

B.　Review of Anatomy on Radiographs

Use those radiographs provided by your instructor.　(These should include radiographs of four basic projections for a skull series, PA Caldwell, AP axial, lateral and submentovertex.)

__　1.　Select good radiographs of the four basic projections for a skull series and identify the following anatomical parts:

- four cranial bones making up the skull cap or calvarium
- petrous pyramids
- mastoid process and tip
- perpendicular plate of ethmoid
- inion
- foramen magnum
- dorsum sellae and posterior clinoid processes
- anterior clinoid processes
- condyles of mandible

- crista galli of ethmoid
- sagittal suture
- lambdoidal suture
- EAM
- clivus
- body of sphenoid (sphenoid sinus)
- foramen ovale
- foramen spinosum
- dens (odontoid process)

C.　Review of Topographical Landmarks and Positioning Lines

Locate the following on another person.

__　1.　Glabella

__　2.　Nasion

__　3.　Vertex

__　4.　Inion

__　5.　TEA

__　6.　EAM

__　7.　Auricle or pinna

__　8.　Angle (gonion)

__　9.　Mental point

__　10.　Acanthion

__　11.　Inner and outer canthi

__　12.　Supraorbital and infraorbital margins

__　13.　Mid-lateral orbital margin

__　14.　Interpupillary line

__　15.　Midsagittal line

__　16.　Glabellomeatal line

__　17.　Orbitomeatal line

__　18.　Infraorbitomeatal line (Reid's base line)

__　19.　Acanthomeatal line

__　20.　Mentomeatal line

__　21.　Glabelloalveolar line

D. Film Critique and Evaluation

Your instructor will provide various radiographs of the basic and optional projections of the cranium as described in this chapter. Some will be of optimal quality radiographs meeting all or most of the evaluation criteria described for each projection in the textbook and/or audio-visuals. Others will be less than optimal quality and several will be unacceptable, requiring a repeat exam. You should evaluate each radiograph as specified below.

Place a check by each of the following when it is completed.

___ 1. Critique each radiograph based on evaluation criteria provided for each projection in the textbook and/or audio-visuals. The following criteria guidelines can be used and checked as each radiograph is evaluated. (Additional checks can be placed to the left for each criteria guideline if more than six radiographs are evaluated.)

       Radiographs   Criteria Guidelines
    1   2   3   4   5   6

— — — — — —   a. Correct film size and correct orientation of part to film?

— — — — — —   b. Correct alignment and/or centering of part to film?

— — — — — —   c. Correct collimation and correct CR location and angle?

— — — — — —   d. Pertinent anatomy well visualized?

— — — — — —   e. Motion?

— — — — — —   f. Optimum exposure; density and/or contrast?

— — — — — —   g. Patient ID information and markers?

___ 2. Based on acceptable variances to criteria factors, determine which of these radiographs are acceptable and which are unacceptable and should have been repeated.

Important: It is important that you have successfully carried out all of the exercises described above before taking the self-test and before going to your instructor for the chapter evaluation exam. If you neglect these exercises, you will not be able to meet all objectives for this chapter and may not receive a passing grade for this course.

Answers to Review Exercise A

1. A.   8
   B.   14

2. A.   Smooth prominence between eyebrows
   B.   Mid-line point at junction of upper lip and nose
   C.   Center of triangle of chin
   D.   A ridge of bone directly above each eye
   E.   Depression or groove above eyebrows
   F.   Depression at the bridge of the nose, or junction of two nasal bones and frontal bone
   G.   The angle or lower posterior portion of jaw or mandible
   H.   Very top or most superior portion of cranium
   I.   The most prominent part of the bump (occipital protuberance) at lower posterior cranium

3. Supraorbital groove

4. A.   Inner canthus
   B.   Outer canthus
   C.   Supraorbital margin
   D.   Infraorbital margin
   E.   Mid-lateral orbital margin

5. A.   External acoustic meatus
   B.   Top of ear attachment
   C.   Supraorbital margin
   D.   Infraorbital margin

6. (a) conical   (b) posteriorly

7. base

8. TEA (top of ear attachment)

9. A.   Midsagittal plane
   B.   Interpupillary line   (IPL)
   C.   Glabellomeatal line   (GML)
   D.   Orbitomeatal line   (OML)
   E.   Infraorbitomeatal line   (IOML)
   F.   Acanthiomeatal line   (AML)
   G.   Mentomeatal line   (MML)
   H.   Glabelloalveolar line   (GAL)

10. Infraorbitomeatal line   (IOML)

11. Interpupillary line (IPL)

12. Midsagittal plane

If you missed more than 10 blanks, you should review this section again in the textbook and/or audio-visuals before continuing.

Answers to Review Exercise B

1. (a) Calvarium
    (b) Frontal bone
    (c) parietal bones
    (d) occipital bone

2. (a) temporal bones
    (b) sphenoid   (c) ethmoid

3. (a) squamous (b) orbital

4. superciliary arch

5. orbital plate

6. parietal bones

7. parietal tubercles (eminences)

8. A. Sutures
    B. Fibrous
    C. Synarthrodial
    D. Immovable
    E. Coronal suture
    F. Sagittal suture
    G. Lambdoidal suture
    H. Squamosal suture
    I. bregma
    J. lambda
    K. fontanels
    L. (a) sphenoid fontanels (b) pterion
    M. (a) mastoid fontanel   (b) asterion
    N. The anterior fontanel
    O. Sutural or Wormian bones

9. occipital

10. foramen magnum

11. (a) lateral condylar portions
    (b) occipital condyles

12. occipito-atlantal

13. A. Coronal suture
    B. Bregma
    C. Squamosal suture
    D. Lambda
    E. Lambdoidal suture
    F. Inion or external occipital
        protuberance
    G. Mastoid fontanel (asterion in adult)
    H. Sphenoid fontanel (pterion in adult)

    I. Frontal eminence
    J. Supraorbital groove
    K. Superciliary arch
    L. Orbital plate of frontal bone

13. *continued*

    M. Nasion
    N. Glabella

14. occipital

15. temporal

16. sphenoid

17. ethmoid

18. squamous

19. (a) zygomatic (b) zygomatic arch

20. temporomandibular

21. styloid

22. (a) mastoid (b) mastoid process

23. (a) petrous pyramids or
        pars petrosa
    (b) petrous ridges

24. (a) sella turcica
    (b) hypophysis (pituitary)

25. (a) dorsum sellae
    (b) posterior clinoid processes

26. (a) anterior clinoid processes
    (b) lesser wings

27. clivus

28. A. lateral pterygoid processes
    B. medial pterygoid processes
    C. pterygoid hamuli

29. (a) foramen rotundum
    (b) foramen ovale
    (c) foramen spinosum

30. seven (all)

31. A. cribriform plate
    B. crista galli
    C. perpendicular plate
    D. labyrinths
    E. (a) nasal conchae (b) turbinates
    F. (a) frontal (b) sphenoid

continued on next page

Answers to Review Exercise B continued

32. A. Zygomatic process
    B. Greater wing of sphenoid
    C. Squamous portion of temporal
    D. Mastoid process
    E. EAM (external acoustic meatus)
    F. Styloid process

    G. Anterior clinoid processes
    H. Posterior clinoid processes
    I. Dorsum sellae
    J. Clivus
    K. Sella turcica

    L. Perpendicular plate of ethmoid
    M. Crista galli of ethmoid
    N. Cribriform plate of ethmoid
    O. Pterygoid process of sphenoid
    P. Pterygoid hamulus of sphenoid

    Q. Crista galli of ethmoid
    R. Cribriform plate of ethmoid
    S. Lesser wing of sphenoid
    T. Greater wing of sphenoid
    U. Foramen ovale of sphenoid
    V. Foramen spinosum of sphenoid
    W. Petrous pyramid of temporal bone
    X. Foramen magnum of occipital bone
    Y. Posterior clinoid process of sphenoid
    Z. Sella turcica of sphenoid
    a. Anterior clinoid processes
    b. Orbital plate of frontal bone

33. (a) parietals (b) sphenoid (c) ethmoid

34. (a) frontal (b) occipital (c) temporal
    (d) sphenoid (e) opposite parietal

35. (a) parietals (b) temporals
    (c) sphenoid (d) atlas (C1)

36. (a) parietal tubercles (eminences)
    (b) 15

37. (a) frontal tuberosity (eminence) of
        forehead
    (b) external occipital protuberance
    (c) 19

38. A. mesocephalic, 47
    B. brachycephalic, greater than 45
        (average ± 54)
    C. dolichocephalic, less than 45
        (average ± 40)

If you missed more than 10 blanks, you should review
this section again in the textbook and/or audio-visuals
before continuing.

Answers to Review Exercise C

1. A. AP axial (Towne)
    B. Lateral
    C. PA or Caldwell
    D. Submentovertex (basilar)

2. Infraorbitomeatal line (IOML)

3. A. Crosswise
    B. Lengthwise
    C. Lengthwise
    D. Lengthwise

4. A. Midsagittal plane - parallel
    B. Interpupillary line - perpendicular

5. A. 2 inches superior to EAM
    B. 3/4 inch anterior and 3/4 inch superior to EAM

6. 7-8

7. A. Mandibular rami
    B. Orbital roofs
    C. Greater or lesser wings of sphenoid
    D. External auditory canals

8. A. Interpupillary
    B. (a) Orbitomeatal (b) Midsagittal
    C. (a) Orbitomeatal (b) Midsagittal

9. A. (a) Caudal (b) 15°
       (c) Orbitomeatal line (OML)
    B. (a) Cephalad (b) 15°
       (c) Orbitomeatal line (OML)
    C. (a) Caudal (b) 30°
       (c) Orbitomeatal line (OML)

10. (a) 30 (b) 37

11. 37° (to IOML) AP axial (Towne), also on the optional PA axial (Haas method) with 25° cephalic angle of CR

12. 30° (to IOML) AP axial

13. (a) sella turcica (b) clivus

14. A. infraorbitomeatal
    B. infraorbitomeatal
    C. (a) anterior (b) petrous pyramids

15. A. (a) Collimated true lateral
       (b) Axial AP
    B. (a) AP axial (b) Submentovertex

16. PA projection (0° CR)

17. Crosstable lateral skull (horizontal beam)

If you missed more than 10 blanks, you should review this section again in the textbook and/or audio-visuals before continuing.

Self-Test

My score = _____ %

Directions: Take this self-test only after completing all the review exercises and laboratory activities in this chapter. Complete directions including grading requirements are described in the front pages of this workbook and in the self-test of Chapter 1.

Test

There are 107 blanks. Each correct blank is worth .9 points. (Spelling is important so correct any misspellings as you grade your test.)

1. The calvarium is formed primarily by the following four cranial bones:

    A. frontal

    B. left parietal

    C. right parietal

    D. occipital

2. The following four cranial bones primarily make up the "floor" of the cranium:

    A. left temporal

    B. right temporal

    C. sphenoid

    D. ethmoid

Matching: (You may use choices more than once)

3. _E_ Auricle

4. _I_ External occipital protuberance

5. _Q_ Smooth prominence between eyebrows

6. _N_ Center of triangle of chin

7. _F_ Groove above eyebrow

8. _B_ Depression at bridge of nose

9. _C_ Top of ear attachment

10. _K_ Medial junction of eyelids near nose

11. _L_ Superior rim of orbit

12. _C_ External landmark corresponding to the petrous ridge

13. _D_ Inferior rim of orbit

14. _G_ Midline point of junction of upper lip and nose

15. _A_ Lower posterior angle of mandible

16. _M_ Lateral portion of orbital rim

17. _D/F_ External landmark corresponding to highest level of facial bone mass

18. _P/O_ Reid's base line

19. _P_ Line between outer canthus and EAM

20. _J_ Most superior portion of cranium

21. _I_ Bump at lower posterior cranium

22. _Z/F_ External landmark corresponding to the level of the floor of cranium

A. Gonion

B. Nasion

C. TEA

D. Infraorbital margin

E. Pinna

F. Supraorbital groove

G. Acanthion

H. EAM

I. Inion

J. Vertex

K. Inner canthus

L. Supraorbital margin

M. Midlateral orbital margin

N. mental point

O. Infraorbitomeatal line

P. Orbitomeatal line

Q. Glabella

Matching: (Match the following with the correct cranial bone)

23. _E_   Lies primarily under floor of cranium   Temporals   (T)

24. _T_   Houses organs of hearing   Parietals   (P)

25. _E_   Crista galli   Frontal   (F)

26. _T_   Styloid process   Occipital   (O)

27. _S_   Sella turcica   Sphenoid   (S)

28. _O_   Inion   Ethmoid   (E)

29. _T_   Mastoid process

30. _S_   Dorsum sellae

31. _S_   Pterygoid process

32. _T_   Zygomatic process

33. _E_   Labyrinths

34. _T_   EAM

35. _E_   Perpendicular plate

36. _E_   Turbinates

37. _O_   Foramen magnum

38. _E_   Cribriform plate

39. _F_   Orbital plate

40. _S_   Lesser wings

41. _F_   Glabella

42. _T_   Petrous pyramids

43. _S_   Clivus

44. _O_   Lateral conylar portions

45. _S_   Foramen rotundum, ovale and spinosum

[Handwritten notes:]

temporals
organs of hearing
styloid process
mastoid process
zygomatic process
EAM
petrous pyramids

frontal
orbital plate
glabella

sphenoid
sella turcica
dorsum sellae
pterygoid process
lesser wings
clivus
foramen rotundum,
ovale, spinosum

ethmoid
lies under floor of
cranium
crista galli
labyrinths
perpendicular plate
turbinates
cribiform plate

occipital
inion
foramen magnum
lateral condylar portions
(occipital condyles)

23

46. Fill in the following from the drawings:

A. glabellomeatal

B. orbitomeatal

C. infraorbitomeatal

D. acanthiomeatal

E. mentomeatal

F. nasion

G. mental point

H. gonion

I. top of ear attachment

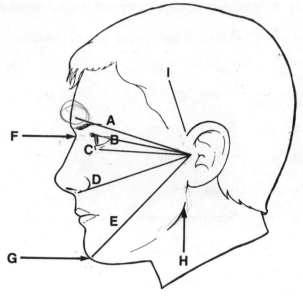

Fig. 11-7

J. frontal bone

K. coronal suture

L. bregma   (anterior fontanel)

M. parietal bone

N. temporal bone

O. squamosal suture

P. lambda   (posterior fontanel)

Q. lambdoidal suture

R. occipital bone

S. asterion   (mastoid fontanel)

T. pterion   (sphenoid fontanel)

U. mastoid tip

V. styloid process

W. ~~ethmoid bone~~   Zygomatic process

X. ~~sphenoid bone~~ greater wing of sphenoid

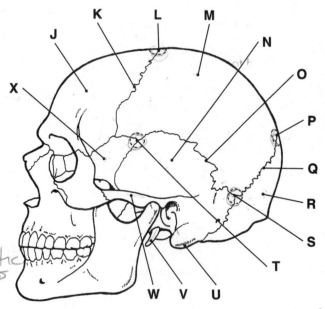

Fig. 11-8

47. Indicate the number of adjoining cranial bones with which each of the following bones articulate.

    A. Frontal   __4__   C. Occipital   __6__   E. Sphenoid __7__

    B. Each parietal __5__   D. Each temporal __3__   F. Ethmoid __2__

48. Complete the following for the correct shape classifications and the degrees of angle between the petrous pyramids and the midsagittal plane:

    A. Average shaped head (a)__mesocephalic__, (b)__47__ degrees

    B. Long narrow head (a)__dolichocephalic__, (b)__40__ degrees

    C. Short broad head (a)__brachycephalic__, (b)__54__ degrees

49. Describe how you would locate the sella turcica from external landmarks.__3/4" anterior__
__+ 3/4" superior to EAM__

50. What are the two lines or planes which should be checked carefully to insure a true lateral skull position?

    A. __midsagittal plane__

    B. __interpupillary line__

51. List the additional terms commonly used to describe the following projections of the skull:

    A. PA, 15° caudal angle __Caldwell__   OML perp.

    B. AP axial __Townes__   30° caudal OML perp

    C. Basilar __Submentovertex__   IOML parallel to film
                                           CR perp to IOML

52. Describe how to locate the correct central ray location for a lateral skull if the entire cranium is to be centered to the film. __2" superior to EAM__

53. How can a person determine by critiquing radiographs if the correct angle of the the central ray was used for the following projections of the cranium:

    A. PA Caldwell? __petrous pyramids fill lower 1/3 of orbits__

    B. AP axial for sella turcica (30° caudal to IOML)? __dorsum sellae + posterior clinoids within shadow of foramen magnum__

    C. AP axial for sella turcica (37° caudal to IOML)? __dorsum sella + posterior clinoids superior to foramen magnum__

    D. Submentovertex? __condyles of mandibles anterior to petrous pyramids__

frontal	parietal	occipital	temporal	sphenoid
parietal	other parietal	L. parietal	one parietal	frontal
parietal	frontal	R. parietal	sphenoid	L. parietal
ethmoid	temporal	L. temporal	occipital	R. parietal
sphenoid	occipital	R. temporal		L. temporal
	sphenoid	sphenoid		R. temporal
ethmoid		(ATLAS)		occipital
frontal				ethmoid
sphenoid				

54. For an AP axial (Towne) projection as part of a routine skull series, which line of the skull should be perpendicular to the film if:

    A. A 30° caudal angle is used? *orbitomeatal line*   *OML*

    B. A 37° caudal angle is used? *infraorbitomeatal line IOML*

55. On a submentovertex projection, the *IOML* line must be parallel to the plane of the film.

56. List the structures best demonstrated on the following cranial projections:

    A. Submentovertex *petrous pyramids, foramen magnum, mastoid processes, foramen ovale, spinosum*

    B. AP axial (30°) *occipital bone, petrous pyramids, foramen magnum dorsum sellae, posterior clinoid processes*

57. What two projections **best** demonstrate the petrous pyramids (ridges)?

    A. *AP axial (Townes)*

    B. *Submentovertex (basilar)*

58. What single projection **best** demonstrates the sella turcica and clivus?

    true lateral, collimated down

59. Which projection **best** demonstrates the internal auditory canals?

    PA projection 0° CR

Answers to Self-Test

1. A. Frontal bone
   B. Right parietal
   C. Left parietal
   D. Occipital bone

2. A. Right temporal
   B. Left temporal
   C. Sphenoid
   D. Ethmoid

3. E; 4. I; 5. Q; 6. N; 7. F;
8. B; 9. C; 10. K; 11. L; 12. C;
13. D; 14. G; 15. A; 16. M; 17. F;
18. O; 19. P; 20. J; 21. I; 22. F.

23. E; 24. T; 25. E; 26. T; 27. S;
28. O; 29. T; 30. S; 31. S; 32. T;
33. E; 34. T; 35. E; 36. E; 37. O;
38. E; 39. F; 40. S; 41. F; 42. T;
43. S; 44. O; 45. S;

46. A. Glabellomeatal line
    B. Orbitomeatal line
    C. Infraorbitomeatal line
    D. Acanthiomeatal line
    E. Mentomeatal line
    F. Nasion
    G. Mental point
    H. Angle or gonion
    I. TEA (top of ear attachment)

    J. Frontal bone
    K. Coronal suture
    L. Bregma
    M. Parietal bone
    N. Temporal bone
    O. Squamosal suture
    P. Lambda
    Q. Lambdoidal suture
    R. Occipital bone
    S. Asterion (mastoid fontanel in newborn)
    T. Pterion (sphenoid fontanel in newborn)
    U. Mastoid tip
    V. Styloid process
    W. Zygomatic process
    X. Greater wing of sphenoid

47. A. 4   C. 6   E. 7
    B. 5   D. 3   F. 2

48. A. (a) Mesocephalic   (b) 47°
    B. (a) Dolichocephalic (b) Approx. 40°
    C. (a) Brachycephalic (b) Approx. 54°

49. 3/4 inch anterior and 3/4 inch superior to EAM

50. A. Midsagittal plane
    B. Interpupillary line (IPL)

51. A. Caldwell
    B. Towne
    C. Submentovertex (SMV)

52. Two inches superior to EAM

53. A. The petrous pyramids should fill lower 1/3 of orbits
    B. Dorsum sellae and posterior clinoids should be visible within the shadow of the foramen magnum
    C. Dorsum sella and posterior clinoids should be just superior to foramen magnum
    D. The condyles of the mandible will be projected just anterior to the petrous pyramids

54. A. Orbitomeatal line (OML)
    B. Infraorbitomeatal line (IOML)

55. Infraorbitomeatal (IOML)

56. A. Petrous pyramids, foramen magnum, mastoid processes, foramen ovale and spinosum
    B. Occipital bone, petrous pyramids, foramen magnum, dorsum sellae and posterior clinoid processes

57. A. AP axial (Towne)
    B. Submentovertex (SMV)

58. True lateral, collimated down

59. PA projection (0° CR)

Chapter 12
Facial Bones

Contributions by: Kathy Martensen, BS, RT(R)

Rationale

Radiography of the facial bones requires a good understanding of the anatomy of these fourteen separate bones. The facial skeleton is difficult to radiograph, not only because of the complexity of these bones, but also because they are situated directly anterior to the very dense cranial structures. For example, how could the maxillary bones comprising the upper jaw be visualized on a frontal projection since the very dense petrous pyramids are located posteriorly and at the same level as these bones? A certain tilt of the head will cause the facial bones to be thrown up just enough so they will be projected on the radiograph slightly higher than the petrous pyramids. Thus it is especially important that you not only know the specific anatomy of the facial bones but also know the relative positions of each specific part of these bones in relationship to other cranial structures.

The orbits or bony cavities of the eye sockets contain small openings for nerves and blood vessels and certain types of pathology or abnormalities involving these openings or foramina can only be diagnosed on radiographs. This again requires a thorough understanding of the shape and structure of the bony orbits in order to be able to direct the central ray precisely through these foramina to visualize them on film. On patients these skeletal structures are covered with skin and other tissues and you must learn and understand this anatomy to the extent that you develop "x-ray sight" and know and be able to "see" and locate these skeletal structures.

It is also very difficult to recognize specific facial and cranial anatomy on radiographs because they often superimpose each other. Even many experienced technologists have difficulty with this. You should take special note of the labeled radiographs in this chapter and learn to look for certain more obvious structures and relate other less obvious structures to them. This will require that you study actual radiographs which are not labeled in the lab and identify all structures identified on the radiographs in the textbook. You will also need to practice each projection and position described in this chapter and evaluate resultant radiographs for proper patient positioning, technical factors, and the visualization of specific needed anatomy.

Chapter Objectives

After you have successfully completed **all** the activities of this unit, you will be able, with at least 80% accuracy, to: (applicable to a written and/or oral examination and demonstration)

___ 1. List the fourteen facial bones (with correct spelling).

___ 2. Identify both on drawings and radiographs, anatomical parts of each facial bone as defined in this chapter in the textbook and/or audio-visuals.

___ 3. Identify the two anatomical names for the "cheek" bone.

___ 4. List the names of specific cranial and facial bones with which each facial bone articulates.

___ 5. Identify the temporomandibular joints (on radiographs) and discriminate between those taken in the open mouth position and those taken in a closed mouth position.

___ 6. Describe the shape and the position of the bony orbits within the skull. Identify the angle formed between the cone-shaped orbits and the orbitomeatal line and between the cone-shaped orbits and the midsagittal plane.

___ 7. List the seven bones making up the orbits and identify which are facial bones and which are cranial bones.

___   8.   Identify on a dry skull each of the seven bones comprising the orbits as well as the three openings of the orbits.

___   9.   List the two basic projections or positions for a routine facial bone series and the optional position for the "floor" of the orbits.

___ 10.   Describe the difference between the routine Waters and the modified Waters positions and describe what anatomical structures are best demonstrated on each.

___ 11.   List the two basic projections or positions taken for a routine zygomatic arch series and the three optional positions or projections.

___ 12.   List the two basic projections or positions for a routine mandible series. Describe the differences in positioning for the axiolateral to best visualize the ramus, the body, or the mentum.

___ 13.   List the optional projections or positions which best demonstrate the following specific parts of the mandible: (1) the upper rami and condyloid processes, (2) the mentum, and (3) the u-shaped outline of the body and mentum.

___ 14.   List the two possible projections for the visualization of the temporomandibular joints and identify the reason for preceding TMJ radiography with routine mandible radiographs. Identify the reason for examining the TMJ's bilaterally and in both the open and closed mouth positions.

___ 15.   Identify the special position commonly used to demonstrate the optic foramen. Describe the positioning line which must be parallel to the central ray, and the degrees of angle between the midsagittal plane and the table top.

___ 16.   Position on a model and/or phantom each of the basic and optional projections as described in the textbook and/or audio-visuals. Include the three different methods for taking each projection which are: (a) on a routine radiographic table, (b) on a vertical head unit or erect table or grid film holder, (c) modifications for severely injured patients.

___ 17   Critique assorted facial, mandibular, and orbital radiographs based on evaluation criteria provided in the textbook and/or audio-visuals.

___ 18.   Discriminate between radiographs which are acceptable and those which are unacceptable due to exposure factors, collimation or positioning errors.

Prerequisite

The prerequisite knowledge required for this chapter is an understanding of radiographic terminology and the principles of exposure, radiation protection, and positioning as defined in Chapter 1. An understanding of the surface landmarks and the localizing lines as described in Chapter 11 as well as the anatomy and positioning of the cranium is essential prior to beginning this chapter on the facial bones. Therefore it is strongly advised that successful completion of both Chapters 1 and 11 be made a mandatory prerequisite for this chapter.

Recommended Supplementary References

The following supplementary references, which are described in more detail in Chapter 1, are listed in a suggested order of importance and value to understand this material.

1. *Merrill's* ..., Vol 2, pp 292-361

2. *Clark's* ..., pp 234-249

3. *Eisenberg* ..., pp 295-313

Learning Exercises

The following review exercises should be completed only after careful study of the associated pages in the textbook and/or audio-visuals as indicated by each exercise.

After completing, check your answers with the answer sheets following these review exercises.

Part I. RADIOGRAPHIC ANATOMY

Review Exercise A   Anatomy of Facial, Nasal, Mandibular, and Orbital Bones

Textbook: pp 341-353
Audio-visuals: Unit 11, slides 1-35
Unit 12, slides 1-12

1. List all of the facial bones and indicate if they are single or paired bones.

Facial bones	Single or Paired
A. maxillae (maxillary)	paired
B. zygomatic (malar)	paired
C. lacrimal	paired
D. nasal bones	paired
E. inferior nasal conchae	paired
F. palatine bones	paired
G. vomer	single
H. mandible	single

2. Complete the following:

A. A second anatomical name for the zygomatic bone is _malar bone_.

B. The largest facial bone is the _mandible_.

C. The largest immovable facial bone is the _maxilla_.

D. Which facial bone assists in forming the mouth, nose, and orbital cavities? _maxilla_

_____.

E. The inferior aspect of the body of the maxilla is called the _alveolar process_.

F. The pointed process of the maxilla located at the acanthion is called the _anterior nasal spine_.

G. The parts of the maxilla which help form the roof of the mouth are the right and left _palatine process_

3. Each maxilla articulates with two cranial bones, (a) _frontal_ and (b) _ethmoid_.

4. List the four separate facial bones which make up the hard palate:

    A. _r. maxilla_   C. _r. palatine_

    B. _l. maxilla_   D. _l. palatine_

5. The zygomatic arch is formed by the (a) _zygomatic_ and (b) _temporal_ bones.

6. The zygomatic prominence is a positioning landmark and refers to the most prominent portion of

    the _zygomatic_ bone.

7. Each nasal bone articulates with which two cranial bones?

    A. _frontal_

    B. _ethmoid_

8. The pair of small facial bones closely associated with the tear ducts are the _lacrimals_ .

9. An incomplete joining of the two palatine processes of the maxillae results in a condition called _____

    cleft palate.

10. The upper teeth are embedded in cavities along the inferior edge of the (a) _alveolar_

    process of the (b) _maxillary_ bones.

11. The large air-filled cavities located in the body of the maxillary bones are called _maxillary_

    sinuses . antrim of Highmore

12. The _frontal_ process of each maxilla projects upward along the lateral border of the nose.

13. The surface landmark located at the point of junction of the frontal bone and the two facial bones forming

    the bridge of the nose is the _nasion_ .

14. List the three pairs of scroll-shaped bones located in the nasal cavity, and identify the cranial or facial
    bone each is associated with.

    Facial or cranial bones

    A. _Superior nasal conchae_   _ethmoid_

    B. _middle nasal conchae_   _ethmoid_

    C. _inferior nasal conchae_   _facial bones_

15. A second name for the above three pairs of bones is _turbinates_ .

16. The superior portion of the bony nasal septum is formed by the (a) _perpendicular pla_

    of the (b) _ethmoid_ , and the inferior portion by the (c) _vomer_ .

17. Identify the anatomy from the labeled drawings and list the name of the bone for which it is a part.

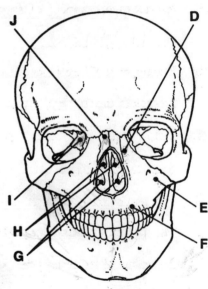

Inferior Surface View   Fig. 12-1

Anatomical Part	Name of facial or cranial bone
A. l. palatine process	l. maxilla
B. l. horizontal process	palatine
C. pterygoid hamulus	sphenoid

D. frontal process   maxilla

E. zygomatic process   maxilla

F. alveolar process   maxilla

G. inferior nasal conchae

H. superior + middle   ethmoid
      nasal conchae

I. lacrimal bone

J. nasal bone

Frontal View   Fig. 12-2

18. The two halves of the mandible join to form a single bone at approximately ___one___ year(s) of age.

19. The Latin word for the chin is ___mentum___.

20. True/False:

     A. __F__ The symphysis of the mandible extends along the complete vertical portion of the mid-anterior mandible. *just the superior portion above the mental protuberance*

     B. __T__ Mental protuberance refers to the lower anterior mandible which projects forward, the center of which is the mental point.

     C. __T__ Symphysis menti is another term for the symphysis of the mandible.

21. Matching:

    A. ___A___ part of mandible   A. coronoid process

    B. ___B___ part of scapula   B. coracoid process

    C. ___A___ part of proximal ulna

22. Label the following drawings of the mandible:

    A. coronoid process

    B. mandibular notch

    C. neck

    D. condyle (head)

    E. condyloid process

    F. ramus

    G. gonion (angle)

    H. body

    I. mentum

    J. alveolar process

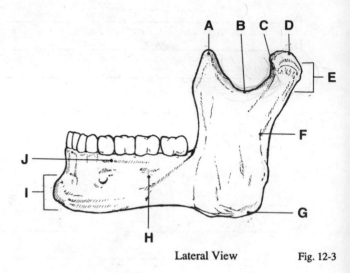

Lateral View   Fig. 12-3

    K. gonion (angle)

    L. mentum

    M. mental point

    N. symphysis menti

    O. mental foramen

    P. ramus

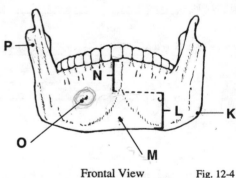

Frontal View   Fig. 12-4

23. A. What is the name of the only synovial/diarthrodial joint of the skull? _freely movable_ TMJ

    B. What movement type(s) is this joint? hinge + gliding

24. There are two types of fibrous/synarthrodial joints of the skull. These are the (a) _non-movable_ sutures of the cranial bones, and the special type of joint involving the teeth and the mandible and maxillae of the subclass termed (b) gomophysis .

25. The condyles of the mandible move (a) _forward_ (forward or backward) to the
(b) _front_ (front or back) edge of the (c) _temporalmandibular_ as the mouth is opened.
fossa

26. Fill in the secondary term for the following parts of the mandible:

    A. Angle _gonion_

    B. Condyle _head_

27. Each orbit is (a) _cone_ shaped and is composed of parts of (b) _7_ (number) bones.

28. With the orbitomeatal line situated parallel with the floor, each orbit projects superiorly at a (a) _30_
    degree angle, and toward the midsagittal plane at (b) _37_ degrees.

29. A small opening termed the _optic foramen_ is located at the _apex_ of each orbit.

30. Fill in the names of the seven bones which form the orbit as indicated in this drawing:

    A. _sphenoid_

    B. _palatine_

    C. _zygomatic_

    D. _ethmoid_

    E. _maxilla_

    F. _lacrimal_

    G. _frontal_

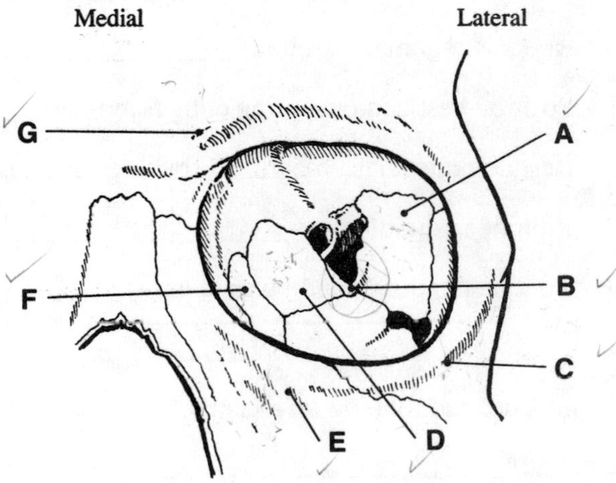

Medial   Lateral

Fig. 12-5

31. Fill in the name of the openings and the one structure (B) in the posterior orbits as indicated in this drawing:

    A. _optic foramen_

    B. _sphenoid strut_

    C. _Superior orbital fissure_

    D. _inferior orbital fissure_

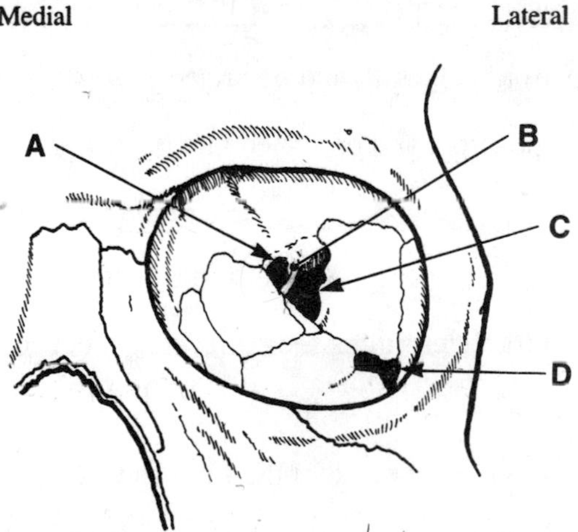

Medial   Lateral

Fig. 12-6

32. Two fractures involving the orbit are known by their descriptive terms as (a) _blow-out_
    and (b) _tripod_ fractures.

Part II. RADIOGRAPHIC POSITIONING

Review Exercise B   Positioning of the Facial and Nasal Bones, Mandible and Orbits

Textbook: pp 354-387
Audio-visuals: Unit 11, slides 36-70
Unit 12, slides 36-53

1. Based on the national survey (as quoted in textbook) list the most frequently performed (basic or routine) positions or projections for the following:

   A. Routine facial bones (a) _lateral_   (b) _PA Waters_ *(parietoacanthial)*

   B. Facial bones on a severely injured trauma patient who cannot be turned into a prone position
   (a) _lateral_ *(crosstable)*   (b) _reverse Waters_ *(acanthioparietal)*

   C. Routine nasal bones (a) _PA Waters_ *(parietoacanthial)*   (b) _laterals_

   D. Routine zygomatic arch (a) _SMV (basilar)_   (b) _PA Waters_

   E. Position best demonstrating optic foramina _Rhese oblique_

   F. Best demonstrates "blow-out" fractures of orbits _modified parietoacanthi_

   G. Routine mandible (a) _axiolateral_ *tube angled 25°*   (b) _PA 0°_

   H. Routine temporomandibular joint (a) _lateral axiolateral oblique_   or (b) _(Law) tube 15° caudal, head turned 15°_
   axiolateral (Schuller)
   tube 25°-30° caudal   mouth opened + closed

2. To prevent head rotation on a lateral facial bone radiograph, the (a) _midsagittal_ plane is aligned (b) _parallel_ to the film and the (c) _interpupillary_ line is aligned to (d) _perpendicular_ to the film.

3. The _parietoacanthial_ projection is another name for the Waters projection. _PA_

4. The petrous ridges should be projected directly below the (a) _maxillary sinuses_ in a Waters position, and projected into the lower half of the maxillary sinuses or below the (b) _inferior orbital rim_ in a modified Waters position.

5. True or false: For a PA Waters, the distance from the tip of the nose to the table top is a good positioning method for determining the correct angle between the orbitomeatal line and the film plane. ___F___

6. In the Waters position, the (a) _OML_ line should form a (b) _37_ degree angle with plane of the film, and a (c) _55_ degree angle in a modified Waters.

7. In the Waters or reverse Waters position, the _mentomeatal_ line should be parallel to the central ray and perpendicular to the plane of the film.

8. In the Waters position, the central ray should exit at the _acanthion_ .

9. In addition to using a small focal spot, a (a) _detail_ film holder should be used to obtain

    optimal detail for a lateral nasal bone radiograph. The kVp range used should be (b) _50-60_ .

10. A good basilar or submentovertex projection requires that the central ray be at right angles to the

    infraorbitomeatal line, which is abbreviated as _IOML_ .

11. For the oblique axial position of the zygomatic arch, the head is turned (a) _15_ degrees toward the side

    being examined, and the midsagittal plane is tilted (b) _15_ degrees.   _Laws_

12. Complete the following for an AP axial projection (Towne position) for the zygomatic arches:

    A. The central ray is directed (a) _30_ degrees (b) _caudal_ (caudal or cephalic) to the

        (c) _OML_ line.

    B. If the infraorbitomeatal line is placed perpendicular to the film, the central ray angulation should be
        IOML

        increased to _37°_ degrees.

13. Indicate the correct central ray location and angulation (indicate as perpendicular if no angle) for the following:

	Central Ray Location	Central Ray Angulation
A. Lateral facial bones	zygoma	perpendicular
B. Reverse Waters	acanthion	perpendicular
C. Lateral nasal bones	½" inferior + posterior to nasion	perpendicular
D. Townes for zygomatic arches	1" superior to glabella	30° caudal to OML
E. Axial obliques for bilateral zygomatic arches	zygomatic arch	perpendicular
F. AP axial projection of mandible _Townes_	glabella	35-40° caudal to OML
G. Axiolateral oblique position of temporomandibular joints	1½" superior to EAM	15° caudal

14. Complete the following for the Rhese position:

    A. As a starting reference position, the three parts of the face which should be touching the table top are

        the _chin_ , _cheek_ and _nose_ . (3 point landing)

    B. The _acanthiomeatal_ line should be perpendicular to the table top and
        parallel to the central ray.

    C. The head should be rotated _37_ degrees from the PA position, which results in a _53_ degree
        angle between the midsagittal plane and the table top.

    D. This position will project the optic foramen into the _lower outer_ quadrant of
        the orbit being examined.

15. What projection or position is most useful in visualizing the condyloid processes and temporomandibular fossae? _AP axial (Townes)_

16. Aligning the _midsagittal_ plane perpendicular to the plane of the film for a PA mandible will prevent rotation.

17. True or false: For the routine PA projection of the mandible, a 15-20 degree caudal angulation is needed. _F_   _CR perpendicular_

18. In the axiolateral projection (oblique position) of the mandible, name that portion of the mandible which would be best demonstrated using the following head rotations.

   A. 30 degree rotation _body_

   B. True lateral (no rotation) _ramus_

   C. 45 degree rotation _mentum_

   tube 25° cephalic

19. Why must the chin be extended when doing the axiolateral projection of the mandible? _to prevent c-spine superimposition_

20. For the axiolateral position a cephalic angle of approximately _25_ degrees is needed to visualize the affected mandible without superimposition of the opposite mandible.

21. For a panorex of the mandible, the (a) _IOML_ line is aligned parallel with the (b) _floor_ .

22. A. The common name for the **axiolateral position** for the temporomandibular joints is the _Schuller_ method.

   B. This position requires the head to be in a true lateral position and the central ray to be angled _25-30_ degrees _caudal_ (caudal or cephalad).

23. A. The **axiolateral oblique position** of the temporomandibular joints is commonly referred to as the _Law_ method.

   B. This requires that the head be rotated (a) _15_ degrees toward the film and the central ray angled (b) _15_ degrees _caudal_ (caudal or cephalad).

Review Exercise C   Laboratory Activity   Textbook: pp 358-387

Part A of this learning activity exercise needs to be carried out in a radiographic laboratory or a general diagnostic room in a radiology department. Parts B and C can be carried out in a classroom or any room where illuminators are available.

A. Positioning Exercise

For this section you need another person or an articulated phantom to act as your patient. Practice the following until you can do each of them accurately and without hesitation. It is important to achieve both accuracy and speed in radiographic positioning. Place a check by each when you have achieved this.

Include the following details as you simulate the basic projections for each exam listed below:

- correct size and type of film holder
- location of central ray and correct centering of part to film
- correct placement of markers
- accurate collimation
- proper use of immobilizing devices when needed
- approximate correct exposure factors
- correct instructions to your patient as you simulate the exposure

__ 1. Erect (with head unit if available or with erect table or other erect grid-film holder), lateral and Waters positions for the facial bones.

__ 2. Severely injured patient who cannot be moved from a supine position on a stretcher. (Spinal injury has been ruled out by crosstable lateral cervical spine). Take a crosstable lateral and a Waters position.

__ 3. Head unit or table top lateral and Waters positions for nasal bones.

__ 4. Head unit or table top submentovertex projection for zygomatic arches.

__ 5. Head unit or table top parieto-orbital projection of the optic foramina.

__ 6. Head unit or table top modified acanthioparietal projection for the orbits.

__ 7. Head unit or table top axiolateral and PA projections of the mandible.

__ 8. Head unit or table top axiolateral oblique position (Law Method) of the temporomandibular joints.

__ 9. Special acanthioparietal projection to demonstrate the "floor" of orbits.

Optional: Using either a sectional or fully articulated phantom, produce a diagnostic radiograph for the following:

__ 1. Parietoacanthial and acanthioparietal projections.

__ 2. Parieto-orbital projection.

__ 3. Axiolateral (oblique) projection of the mandible.

__ 4. Axiolateral oblique position (Law Method) of the temporomandibular joints.

B. Review of Anatomy on Radiographs

Use those radiographs provided by your instructor. (These should include an assortment of radiographs, such as a lateral, parietoacanthial, PA Caldwell, submentovertex, Rhese oblique, Law, and Schuller methods.)

___ 1. Identify the following anatomical parts on selected accurately positioned radiographs.

- greater wings of the sphenoid
- sella turcica
- mandible
- maxillae
- zygomatic arches
- orbital rim
- optic foramen
- temporomandibular joints
- coronoid process of mandible
- petrous ridges

- orbital roofs
- zygoma
- inferior rim of orbit
- nasal septum
- anterior nasal spine
- nasal bones
- mandibular rami
- condyloid processes of mandible
- temporomandibular fossae

C. Review of Topographical Landmarks and Positioning Lines
(as used for facial, mandibular, and orbital bone positioning.)

Locate the following on another person.

___ 1. Midsagittal plane

___ 2. Interpupillary line

___ 3. Zygoma

___ 4. Outer canthus

___ 5. EAM

___ 6. Mentomeatal line

___ 7. Acanthion

___ 8. Orbitomeatal line

___ 9. Infraorbitomeatal line

___ 10. Glabelloalveolar line

___ 11. Mandibular symphysis

___ 12. Angles of the mandible

___ 13. Glabella

___ 14. Zygomatic arch

___ 15. Zygomatic prominence

___ 16. Three point landing for Rhese method

___ 17. Superciliary arch

C. Film Critique and Evaluation

Your instructor will provide various radiographs of the basic and optional projections of the facial bones as described in this chapter. Some will be optimal quality radiographs meeting all or most of the evaluation criteria described for each projection in the textbook and/or audio-visuals. Others will be less than optimal quality and several will be unacceptable, requiring a repeat exam. You should evaluate each radiograph as specified below.

Place a check by each of the following when it is completed.

___ 1. Critique each radiograph based on evaluation criteria provided for each projection in the textbook and/or audio-visuals. The following criteria guidelines can be used and checked as each radiograph is evaluated. (Additional checks can be placed to the left for each criteria guideline if more than six radiographs are evaluated.)

      Radiographs   Criteria Guidelines
   1 2 3 4 5 6

___ ___ ___ ___ ___ ___   a. Correct film size and correct orientation of part to film?

___ ___ ___ ___ ___ ___   b. Correct alignment and/or centering of part to film or portion of film being used?

___ ___ ___ ___ ___ ___   c. Correct collimation and CR location?

___ ___ ___ ___ ___ ___   d. Pertinent anatomy well visualized?

___ ___ ___ ___ ___ ___   e. Motion?

___ ___ ___ ___ ___ ___   f. Optimum exposure; density and/or contrast?

___ ___ ___ ___ ___ ___   g. Patient ID information and markers?

___ 2. Based on acceptable variances to criteria factors, determine which of these radiographs are acceptable and which are unacceptable and should have been repeated.

Important: It is important that you have successfully carried out all of the exercises described above before taking the self-test and before going to your instructor for the chapter evaluation exam. If you neglect these exercises, you will not be able to meet all the objectives for this chapter and may not receive a passing grade for this course.

Answers to Review Exercise A

1. A. Maxillae, paired
    B. Zygomatic, paired
    C. Lacrimal, paired
    D. Nasal, paired
    E. Inferior nasal conchae, paired
    F. Palatine, paired
    G. Vomer, single
    H. Mandible, single

2. A. malar
    B. mandible
    C. maxillary bones or maxillae
    D. Maxillary bones or maxillae
    E. alveolar process
    F. anterior nasal spine
    G. palatine process

3. (a) frontal   (b) ethmoid

4. A. Right maxilla
    B. Left maxilla
    C. Right palatine bone
    D. Left palatine bone

5. (a) zygomatic   (b) temporal

6. zygomatic

7. A. Frontal
    B. Ethmoid

8. lacrimal

9. cleft palate

10. (a) alveolar   (b) maxillary

11. maxillary sinuses

12. frontal

13. nasion

14. A. Superior nasal cochae   ethmoid
    B. Middle nasal conchae   ethmoid
    C. Inferior nasal conchae   inferior nasal
        conchae

15. turbinates

16. (a) perpendicular plate (b) ethmoid
    (c) vomer

17. A. Left palatine process   maxilla
    B. Left horizontal process   palatine
    C. Pterygoid hamulus   sphenoid

     D. Frontal process   maxilla
     E. Zygomatic process   maxilla
     F. Alveolar process   maxilla
     G. Inferior nasal conchae
     H. Middle nasal conchae   ethmoid
     I. Lacrimal bone
     J. Nasal bone

18. one

19. mentum or mental

20. A. false (just the superior portion
        above the mental protuberance)
    B. true
    C. true

21. A. A
    B. B
    C. A

22. A. Coronoid process
    B . Mandibular Notch
    C. Neck
    D. Condyle (head)
    E. Condyloid process
    F. Ramus
    G. Angle (gonion)
    H. Body
    I. Mental protuberance
    J. Alveolar process

    K. Angle (gonion)
    L. Mental protuberance
    M. Mental point
    N. Symphysis of mandible (symphysis
        menti)
    O. Mental foramen
    P. Ramus

23. A. Temporomandibular joint (TMJ)
    B. Hinge and gliding (two movement types)

24. (a) sutures   (b) gomphosis

25. (a) forward   (b) front
    (c) temporomandibular fossa

26. A. Gonion
    B. Head

27. (a) cone   (b) seven

28. (a) 30   (b) 37

29. optic foramen,   apex

Answers to Review Exercise A continued

30. A. Sphenoid
     B. Palatine
     C. Zygomatic
     D. Ethmoid
     E. Maxilla
     F. Lacrimal
     G. Frontal

31. A. Optic foramen
     B. Sphenoid strut
     C. Superior orbital fissure
     D. Inferior orbital fissure

32. (a) blow-out   (b) tripod

If you missed more than 20 blanks, you should review this section again in the textbook and/or audio-visuals before continuing.

Answers to Review Exercise B

1. A. (a) lateral (b) parietoacanthial
    B. (a) crosstable lateral (b) acanthioparietal
    C. (a) lateral (b) parietoacanthial
    D. (a) submentovertex (b) parietoacanthial
    E. parieto-orbital (Rhese)
    F. modified parietoacanthial
    G. (a) axiolateral oblique (b) PA
    H. (a) axiolateral oblique (Law)
        (b) axiolateral (Schuller)

2. (a) midsagittal (b) parallel (c) interpupillary
    (d) perpendicular

3. parietoacanthial

4. (a) maxillary sinuses
    (b) inferior orbital rim

5. false (too much variance on length of noses)

6. (a) orbitomeatal (b) 37 (c) 55

7. mentomeatal

8. acanthion

9. (a) detail screen (b) 50-60

10. infraorbitomeatal, IOML

11. (a) 15 (b) 15

12. A. (a) 30 (b) caudal (c) orbitomeatal
    B. 37

13. A. zygoma   perpendicular
    B. acanthion   perpendicular
    C. .5 inches inferior and
        posterior to nasion   perpendicular
    D. 1 inch superior to   30 degrees caudal
        glabella   to OML
    E. zygomatic arch   perpendicular
    F. glabella   35 to 40 degrees
                                            caudal to OML
    G. 1.5 superior to   15 degrees
        upside EAM   caudal

14. A. chin, nose and cheek
    B. acanthiomeatal
    C. 37, 53
    D. lower outer

15. AP axial projection (Towne)

16. midsagittal

17. false (CR is perpendicular)

18. A. body
    B. ramus
    C. mentum

19. prevent superimposition of cervical spine

20. 25

21. (a) infraorbitomeatal line (b) floor

22. A. Schuller

    B. 25-30 caudal

23. A. Law

    B. (a) 15 (b) 15 caudal

If you missed more than 14 blanks, you should review this section again in the textbook and/or audio-visuals before continuing.

Self-Test

My score = _____ %

Directions: Take this self-test only after completing all the review exercises and laboratory activities in this chapter. Complete directions including grading requirements are described in the front pages of this workbook and in the self-test of Chapter 1.

Test

There are 112 blanks. Each correct blank is worth .9 point. (Spelling is important so correct any misspellings as you grade your test.)

1. Identify the labeled anatomy and list the name of which bone it is a part where indicated:

Anatomical Part	Name of Facial or Cranial Bone
A. frontal bone	
B. greater wing	sphenoid
C. zygomatic process	temporal
D. condyle (head)	mandible
E. ramus	mandible
F. body	mandible
G. alveolar process	maxilla
H. zygomatic (malar) bone	
I. anterior nasal spine	maxilla
J. frontal process	maxilla
K. lacrimal bone	
L. nasion	

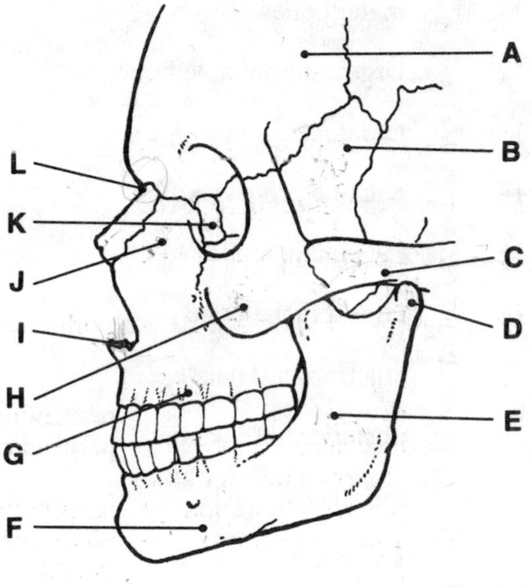

Fig. 12-7

2. Fill in the names of three openings of the orbits.

A. Superior orbital fissure

B. inferior orbital fissure

C. optic foramen

3. The small <u>root of bone</u> forming the lateral wall of the optic canal, important in radiology, is the _____ sphenoid strut .

Matching: Match the correct facial bone(s) for the following:

4. __F__ bony nasal septum *Vomer*

5. __A__ frontal process *A*

6. __D__ nasion *D*

7. __A__ maxillary sinuses *A*

8. __A__ assists in formation of the three *A* facial cavities

9. __A+E__ alveolar process *A/E*

10. __A__ zygomatic process *A*

11. __B__ malar bones *B*

12. __A__ largest immovable bone *A*

13. __C__ tear ducts *c*

14. __A__ palatine processes *A*

15. __B__ zygomatic arches *B*

16. __E__ largest facial bone *E*

17. __A__ anterior hard palate *A*

18. __G__ posterior hard palate *G*

19. __H__ turbinates *H*

20. __A__ anterior nasal spine *A*

21. __E__ coronoid process *E*

A. Maxillae

B. Zygomatic bones

C. Lacrimal bones

D. Nasal bones

E. Mandible

F. Vomer

G. Palatine bones

H. Inferior nasal conchae

22. The two common types of fractures involving the orbits are:

A. blow-out

B. tripod

blow-out - floor of the orbit

tripod - zygomatic bone + three connections -
maxilla
temporal
frontal

23.   Identify the names of the bones and the openings as labeled on this drawing of the orbit.

   A. optic foramina

   B. frontal

   C. sphenoid strut

   D. superior orbital fissure

   E. sphenoid

   F. zygomatic

   G. inferior orbital fissure

   H. palatine

   I. maxilla

   J. lacrimal

   K. ethmoid

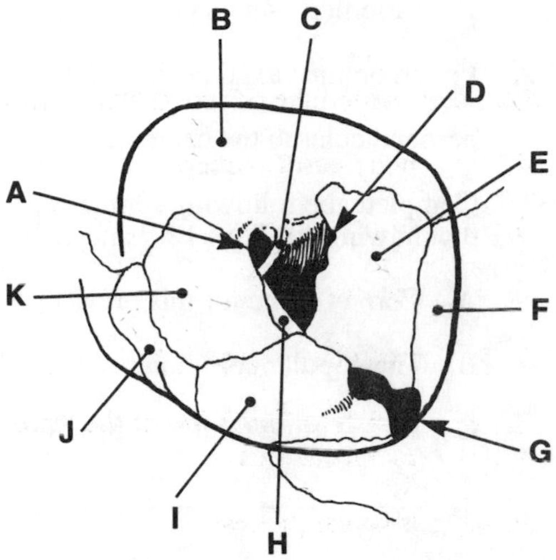

Medial   Lateral
                                Fig. 12-8

24.   What two structures make up the bony nasal septum?

   A. vomer

   B. perpendicular plate of ethmoid

25.   What is the name of the projection describing the PA Waters position? parietoacanthial

26.   What anatomical part is best demonstrated on the following?

   A. Waters maxillary area

   B. Modified Waters floor of orbits

   C. Rhese position optic foramen

27.   What two anatomical parts or areas should be superimposed in an optimal modified parietoacanthial
       projection? (a) petrous ridges and (b) lower half of maxillary sinuses area just below infraorbital rim

28.   What two anatomical parts or areas should be superimposed in an optimal Waters position?

   (a) petrous ridges and (b) area just below maxillary sinuses

29.   List the name of the position taken in place of the Waters for the patient with possible spinal injuries who
       cannot be turned prone, and describe how it would be done. reverse Waters acanthioparietal
       pat. supine, CR parallel to mentomeatal line

30.   How can rotation be determined on a radiograph taken in either the Waters or modified Waters positions?

   equal distance from nasal septum to outer skull
   margin, or equal distance from lateral
   orbital margins to lateral margins of skull

31. List the degrees of angle between the orbitomeatal line and the plane of the film for:

    A. Waters position _____37_____ degrees

    B. Modified Waters position _____55_____ degrees

    Mentomeatal line ⊥

    IOML - pg

32. For an oblique axial position for the right zygomatic arch, the ___infraorbital___ line is
    (aves)
    perpendicular to the central ray and the head is rotated ___15___ degrees toward the affected side.

33. Complete the following for the special projection to demonstrate the optic foramina as demonstrated by the drawings in Figs. 12-9 and 12-10.

    A. Correct name for this projection ___parieto-orbital___

    B. The popular common name for this projection ___Rhese method___

    C. As a starting reference position, name the three "points" which should be touching the table.

    ___chin___, ___cheek___, and ___nose___

    Fill in the correct angles from the following drawings:

    D. _____30_____ degrees

    E. _____37_____ degrees

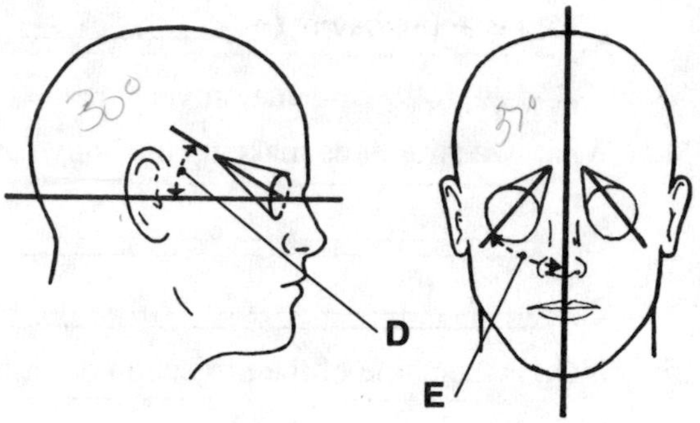

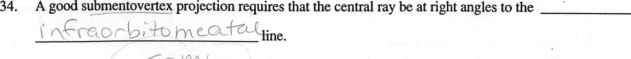

Fig. 12-9

    F. _____37_____ degrees

    G. _____53_____ degrees

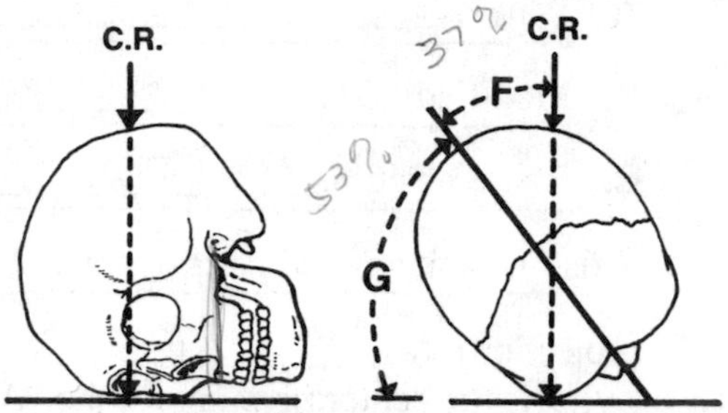

Fig. 12-10

    H. Name the positioning line which is parallel to the central ray. ___acanthiomeatal line___

    I. The position demonstrated in Fig. 12-9 will demonstrate the (a) ___right___ (right or left) *PA - dow*
       AP - up
       optic foramen within the (b) ___lower outer___ quadrant of the orbit.

34. A good submentovertex projection requires that the central ray be at right angles to the _____
    ___infraorbitomeatal___ line.
    (___IOML___)

35. Complete the following for an AP axial projection (Townes) for the zygomatic arches:

  A. Central ray should enter head at ___1" superior to glabella___.

  B. Tuck the patient's chin, bringing the ___orbitomeatal OML___ line perpendicular to the film.

  C. The central ray should be angled _30_ degrees ___caudal___ (caudal or cephalad).

36. The correct central ray location for a reverse Waters is to the ___acanthion___.

37. In a Waters position, the ___mentomeatal___ line should be perpendicular to the plane of the film.

38. A. The triangular area of the mandible projecting anteriorly is called the ___mental protuberance___.

  B. The center of this triangle is the ___mental point___.

39. The (a) ___condyle (head)___ of the mandible fits into the (b) ___temporomandibular___ fossa of the (c) ___temporal___ bone to form the (d) ___temporomandibular___ joint which is abbreviated (e) ___TMJ___. ___synovial / diarthrodial___

40. Fill in the following anatomy:

  A. ___coronoid process___

  B. ___mandibular notch___

  C. ___neck___

  D. ___condyle or head___

  E. ___condyloid process___

  F. ___ramus___

  G. ___body___

  H. ___gonion or angle___

  I. ___alveolar process___

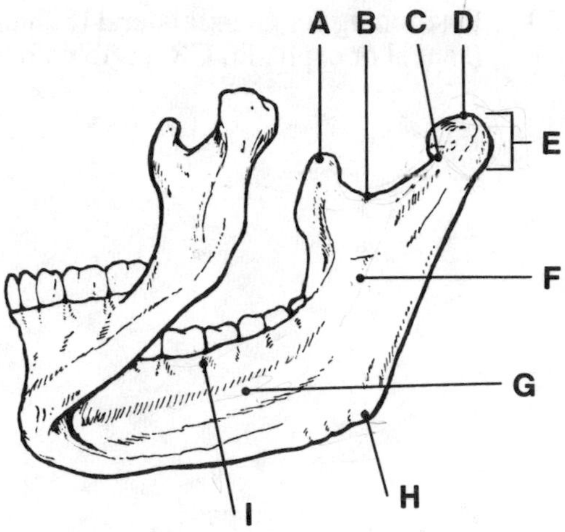

Fig. 12-11

41. What is the centering point for the PA projection of the mandible? ___junction of lips___

42. Describe how you would position for an axiolateral oblique mandible for the right mandibular body.
___patient's head right lateral, turn 30° toward film + extend chin___

43. For an axiolateral or oblique mandible the central ray is angled _25_ degrees ___cephalic___ (caudal or cephalad).

44. What is the name of the basic projection which demonstrates the mandibular rami and lateral portion of body? ___PA projection___

45. What projection best visualizes the upper rami and condyloid processes of the mandible?

     AP axial (Townes)

46. Name the two basic positions/projections for radiographing the temporomandibular joints: (Include the common name for each.)

     A. *axiolateral oblique* (*Law*)

     B. *axiolateral* (*Schuller*)

47. Why are temporomandibular radiographs taken bilaterally and in both the open and closed mouth position?

     to compare right + left sides, to demonstrate movement of mandibular condyle within the temporomandibular fossa.

48. Should the open and closed positions be attempted in TMJ radiography if the patient has a possible fracture of the mandible? *no*

49. Positioning for the axiolateral oblique (Law) position requires a double *15* degree angle. (Head rotation and CR angle.)

50. Positioning for an axiolateral (Schuller) position requires a *25-30* degree *caudal* (caudal or cephalic) CR angle with the head in a true lateral position.

Answers to Self-Test

1. A. Frontal bone
    B. Greater wing — sphenoid
    C. Zygomatic process — temporal
    D. Condyle (head) — mandible
    E. Ramus — mandible
    F. Body — mandible
    G. Alveolar process — maxilla
    H. Zygomatic (malar) bone
    I. Anterior nasal spine — maxilla
    J. Frontal process — maxilla
    K. Lacrimal bone
    L. Nasion

2. A. Superior orbital fissure
    B. Inferior orbital fissure
    C. Optic foramen

3. sphenoid strut

4. F
5. A
6. D
7. A
8. A
9. A and E
10. A
11. B
12. A
13. C
14. A
15. B
16. E
17. A
18. G
19. H
20. A
21. E

22. A. Blow-out
    B. Tripod

23. A. Optic foramina
    B. Frontal
    C. Sphenoid strut
    D. Superior orbital fissure
    E. Sphenoid
    F. Zygomatic
    G. Inferior orbital fissure
    H. Palatine
    I. Maxilla
    J. Lacrimal
    K. Ethmoid

24. A. Vomer
    B. Perpendicular plate of ethmoid

25. Parietoacanthial

26. A. maxillary area
    B. floor of orbits
    C. optic foramen

27. (a) petrous ridges (b) area just below infra-orbital rim, or inferior half of maxillary sinuses

28. (a) petrous ridges (b) area just below maxillary sinuses

29. Reverse Waters, patient supine with the central ray directed parallel with the mentomeatal line

30. Equal distance from nasal septum to the outer skull margin on each side, or equal distance from the lateral orbital margins to the lateral margins of the skull

31. A. 37
    B. 55

32. infraorbital, 15

33. A. Parieto-orbital
    B. Rhese method
    C. chin, cheek, nose
    D. 30
    E. 37
    F. 37
    G. 53
    H. acanthiomeatal line
    I. (a) right (b) lower outer

34. infraorbitomeatal

35. A. 1 inch superior to glabella
    B. orbitomeatal
    C. 30, caudal

36. acanthion

37. mentomeatal

38. A. mental protuberance
    B. mental point

39. (a) condyle (head) (b) temporomandibular (c) temporal (d) temporomandibular (e) TMJ

40. A. Coronoid process
    B. Mandibular notch
    C. Neck
    D. Condyle or head
    E. Condyloid process
    F. Ramus
    G. Body
    H. Gonion or angle
    I. Alveolar process

Answers to Self-Test continued

41. junction of lips

42. Start with patient's head lateral with the right
     side toward film, from this position turn face
     30 degrees toward film and extend chin

43. 25, cephalad

44. PA projection

45. AP axial (Towne)

46. A. Axiolateral oblique (Law)
     B. Axiolateral (Schuller)

47. To compare right and left sides and to
     demonstrate movement of the mandibular
     condyle within the temporomandibular fossa.

48. no (may result in fracture displacement)

49. 15

50. 25 to 30, caudal

Chapter 13

Paranasal Sinuses, Mastoids and Temporal Bone

Contributions by: Kathy Martensen, BS, RT(R)

Rationale

This chapter covers the paranasal sinuses, mastoids and the complex temporal bone. The difficulty level of this chapter is similar to that of the previous two chapters on the skull and facial bones. All students and technologists should master this material because they will encounter most of these examinations as technologists working in a general hospital or clinic.

Radiographs of the paranasal sinuses are common examinations similar to that of the skull and facial bones. The mastoids and temporal bones however are somewhat of a rarity in many departments, which makes it even more important that all students and technologists understand the anatomy and positioning of these body parts well enough to be competent in radiographing these when necessary.

This chapter is especially well suited for in-service training for those technologists and students who do not have much exposure to these more specialized procedures involving the skull.

Chapter Objectives

After you have successfully completed **all** the activities of this chapter, you will be able, with at least 80% accuracy, to: (applicable to a written and/or oral examination and demonstration)

___ 1. Locate the four groups of paranasal sinuses on either frontal or lateral view radiographs and list the usual number of sinuses in each group.

___ 2. Describe the three main portions of the temporal bones.

___ 3. Identify on drawings the location and extent of the three divisions of the ear and give the name or names for each structure of the three portions of the ear.

___ 4. Describe the shape and relative positions of the three ossicles of the middle ear as seen from both a frontal and lateral view.

___ 5. Identify the distances between various structures of the ear and the distances from the table top to these structures in both frontal and lateral positions.

___ 6. Given any two structures of the petrous and mastoid portions of the temporal bone, be able to determine which is located more lateral or which is more posterior.

___ 7. List the four basic projections or positions for a routine paranasal sinus series.

___ 8. List the three basic projections or positions for a routine mastoid series as well as the two optional projections.

___ 9. List the two projections or positions used to best visualize the petrous portion of the temporal bone in addition to routine skull radiography.

___ 10. Position on a model and/or phantom each of the basic and optional projections as described in the textbook and/or audiovisuals. Include the different methods for taking each projection which are: (a) on a routine radiographic table, and (b) on a vertical head unit or erect table or grid film holder.

___ 11. Critique assorted paranasal sinus, mastoid, and temporal bone radiographs based on evaluation criteria provided in the textbook and/or audiovisuals.

___ 12. Discriminate between radiographs which are acceptable and those which are unacceptable because of exposure factors, collimation or positioning errors.

Prerequisite

The minimum prerequisite knowledge requirement for this chapter is an understanding of radiographic terminology and principles as defined in Chapter 1, and the anatomy and positioning of the cranium and facial bones as described in Chapters 11 and 12. It is strongly advised that successful completion of Chapters 1, 11, and 12 be made mandatory prerequisites for this chapter.

Recommended Supplementary References

The following supplementary references, which are described in more detail in Chapter 1, are listed in a suggested order of importance and value to understand this material.

1. *Merrill's ...*, Vol 2, pp 364-447

2. *Clark's ...*, pp 214-232

Learning Exercises

The following review exercises should be completed only after careful study of the associated pages in the textbook and/or audio-visuals as indicated by each exercise.

After completing, check your answers with the answer sheets following these review exercises.

Part I. RADIOGRAPHIC ANATOMY

Review Exercise A   Anatomy of paranasal sinuses, mastoids and temporal bone.

Textbook: pp 389-397
Audio-visuals: Unit 12, slides 13-34

1. Identify the paranasal sinuses from the following drawings: (Include the usual number of sinuses in each group where indicated.)

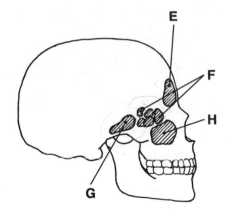

Fig. 13-1

<u>Sinuses</u>	<u>Usual Number</u>
A. frontal	2
B. ethmoid	many
C. sphenoid	1 or 2
D. maxillary	2

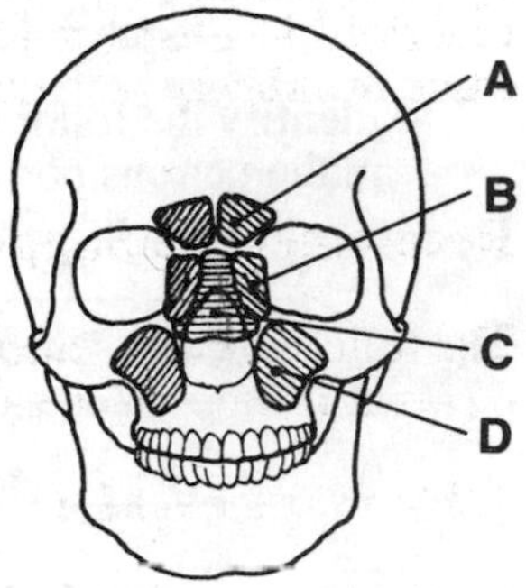

E. frontal

F. ethmoid

G. sphenoid

H. maxillary

Fig. 13-2

2. What is the older term sometimes found in literature referring to the maxillary sinuses? _____

Antrum of Highmore

3. The communication between each maxillary sinus and the respective nasal cavity is relatively superior (inferior or superior) to the cavity itself.

4. The air cells of the ethmoid sinuses are contained in the (a) labyrinths of the (b) ethmoid bone.
    (lateral masses)

271

5. The sphenoid sinus lies in the (a) _body_ of the (b) _sphenoid_ bone.

6. True or false:

A. _F_ The frontal sinuses usually have some air in them at birth but the maxillary sinuses seldom do.
   maxillary sinuses only ones at birth

B. _T_ The frontal sinuses are not always paired and often are not symmetrical in shape.

C. _F_ The ethmoid sinuses are usually comprised of two groups. *three - anterior, middle, posterior*

D. _T_ Both the maxillary and ethmoid sinuses communicate with the nasal cavity.

E. _T_ A horizontal beam radiograph of the sphenoid sinus may be of assistance in diagnosing a basal skull fracture.

F. _F_ It is important to take sinus radiographs in an erect position because fluid will remain trapped in the frontal sinuses in this position. *maxillary sinuses*

G. _T_ Infections originating in the upper teeth may pass up into the maxillary sinuses.

7. Identify the following anatomy on the labeled drawings of the organs of hearing and equilibrium located in the petrous portion of the temporal bones:

A. auricle (pinna)
B. external acoustic meatus
C. tympanic membrane *drum crest or spur*
D. auditory ossicles
E. epitympanic recess (attic)
F. osseous labyrinth *semicircular canals*
G. internal auditory meatus
H. tympanic cavity
I. cochlea
J. eustachian tube (auditory tube)
K. styloid process
L. mastoid process (tip)

M. malleus
N. incus
O. stapes

Lateral   A B C E D F G   Medial

H
I
J
L   K

Frontal View   Fig. 13-3

M N O

Lateral   Medial

Auditory Ossicles, Frontal View   Fig. 13-4

7. *continued*

P. external acoustic meatus

Q. stapes

R. incus

S. malleus

Anterior or Posterior

T. anterior

U. posterior

Auditory Ossicles, Lateral View   Fig. 13-5

8. Identify the labeled parts of this drawing of the osseous (bony) labyrinth:

A. posterior semicircular canal

B. lateral semicircular canal

C. superior semicircular canal

D. oval window (vestibular window)

E. vestibule

F. cochlea

G. round window (cochlear window)

Anterior or Posterior

H. anterior

I. posterior

Lateral View   Fig. 13-6

9. The two main portions of the internal ear are:

A. osseous (bony) labyrinth   B. membranous labyrinth

10. That portion of the internal ear housing the organs of hearing is the (a) cochlea , and

housing the organs of equilibrium is the (b) semicircular canals

11. Fill in the following distances on an average shaped, mesocephalic skull.

Anterior-posterior measurements with OML perpendicular to table top:

A. Back of head to mid EAM   10   cm.

B. Anterior cochlea to posterior ear structures   1-1.5 cm.

Lateral measurements: (To side away from table top)

C. Table top to external opening of external acoustic meatus   14   cm.

D. Table top to distal internal auditory meatus   9   cm.

E. Distance from external opening of external acoustic meatus to internal acoustic meatus   5   cm.

Part II. RADIOGRAPHIC POSITIONING

Review Exercise B   Positioning of the Paranasal Sinuses, Mastoids, and Temporal Bones

Textbook: pp 398-409
Audio-visuals: Unit 12, slides 54-73

1. Which paranasal sinuses are **best** demonstrated on the following projections/positions?

    A. PA Caldwell _frontal_

    B. Waters _maxillary_

    C. Lateral _sphenoid_

2. Why must sinus radiography be done erect and with a <u>horizontal beam</u>? _to show_
    fluid levels   air-fluid levels

3. List the four basic or routine projections or positions most commonly performed for paranasal sinuses:
    (Include common name where applicable.)

    A. _lateral_ (_____)

    — B. _PA_ (_Caldwell_) _15°_

    — C. _parietoacanthial_ (_Waters_)

    D. _submentovertex_ (_basilar   SMV_)

4. Which <u>optional</u> projection is most common for the paranasal sinuses? _axial transoral_
    (open-mouth Waters) —

5. List the cranial positioning line which should be perpendicular to the plane of the film on the following
    paranasal sinus projections or positions: (Include initials where indicated.)

    A. Lateral position _interpupillary_ (_IPL_)

    B. PA (Caldwell) projection _orbitomeatal_ (_OML_)

    C. Parietoacanthial projection (Waters) _mentomeatal_ (_MML_)

6. Where should the film be centered for the following paranasal sinus projections and positions?

    Waters
    A. Parietoacanthial _acanthion_

    B. PA (Caldwell) _nasion_

    C. Lateral _midway btw. outer canthus and EAM_

7. Evidence for a basilar skull <u>fracture</u> may be supported by air-fluid levels demonstrated in the _sphenoid_
    sinuses.

8. The two most common **basic** or **routine** projections/positions for the <u>mastoids</u> are: (Include the common
    name where indicated.)

    A. _axiolateral_ (_Law_)

    B. _anterior oblique_ (_Stenvers_)
        posterior profile

9. The two most common **optional** projections/positions for the mastoids are: (Include common names.)

    A. ___AP axial_____ (_Towne_____)

    B. _Axioposterior oblique_ (_Mayer_____)

10. Why must the pinna of the ear be taped forward when examining the mastoid air cells? _to_____ _prevent it from superimposing_

11. In the posterior profile (Stenvers) position with a mesocephalic skull, the petrous pyramid of interest is placed (a) _parallel_ (parallel or perpendicular) to the plane of the film by rotating the head (b) _45_ degrees to the plane of the film. The central ray is angled (c) _12_ degrees (d) _cephalic_ (caudal or cephalic). _CR 1" anterior to EAM down_

12. In the posterior profile position (Stenvers) the _down-side_ (down-side or up-side) petrous pyramid is being radiographed.

13. Whenever radiographing mastoids it is necessary to perform a _bilateral_ (unilateral or bilateral) examination.

14. In the axiolateral oblique (Law) position the (a) _down-side_ (up-side or down-side) is the area of interest. The cassette centering point (anatomical part to the center of the film) is (b) _____ _mastoid tip 1" posterior to EAM_

15. Which of the two basic mastoid projections/positions best demonstrates the bony labyrinth, tympanic cavity and internal acoustic canal? _AP axial_ _posterior profile position_ (_Townes_ _Stenvers_)

16. The two most common basic projections/positions for the petrous pyramids are: (Include common names.)

    A. ___AP axial_____ (_Townes_____)

    B. _submentovertex_ (_basilar_____)

17. A special radiographic method or procedure to best visualize the delicate structures of the middle and internal ears which are surrounded and superimposed by dense bone structure is termed _tomography_

18. Select the structure which is the more anterior of the two.

    A. Ossicles or semicircular canals ___ossicles_____

    B. Internal acoustic canal or tympanic cavity _tympanic cavity_

    C. Mastoid antrum or ossicles ___ossicles_____

19. Select the structure which is the more lateral of the two.

    A. Ossicles or semicircular canals _ossicles_____

    B. Internal acoustic canal or cochlea _cochlea_____

    C. External acoustic canal or vestibule _EAM_____

Part A of this learning activity exercise needs to be carried out in a radiographic laboratory or general diagnostic room in a radiology department. Parts B and D can be carried out in a classroom or any room where illuminators are available.

A. Positioning Exercise

For this section you need another person or an articulated phantom to act as your patient. Practice the following until you can do each of them accurately and without hesitation. It is important to achieve both accuracy and speed in radiographic positioning. Place a check by each when you have achieved this.

Include the following details as you simulate the basic projections for each exam listed below:

- correct size and type of film holder
- location of central ray and correct centering of part to film
- correct placement of markers
- accurate collimation
- proper use of immobilizing devices when needed
- approximate correct exposure factors
- correct instructions to your patient as you simulate the exposure

___ 1. Erect (with head unit if available or with erect table or other grid-film holder), Lateral, PA Caldwell, Parietoacanthial, and Submentovertex projections for paranasal sinuses.

___ 2. Head unit or table top axiolateral oblique and posterior profile projections for mastoids.

___ 3. Head unit or table top AP axial and submentovertex projections for petrous pyramids.

Optional: Using either a sectional or fully articulated phantom, produce a diagnostic radiograph for the above projections/ positions for the paranasal sinuses, mastoids and petrous pyramids.

B. Review of Anatomy on Radiographs

Use those radiographs provided by your instructor. (These should include an assortment of radiographs, such as a lateral, PA Caldwell, Waters, Axiolateral Oblique, Posterior Profile, and Submentovertex.)

1. Identify the following anatomical parts on selected accurately positioned radiographs.

- sphenoid sinuses
- frontal sinus
- ethmoid sinuses
- maxillary sinuses
- sella turcica
- orbital roofs
- nasal fossae
- mastoid air cells
- petrous ridges
- bony labyrinth
- tympanic cavity
- internal auditory canal
- external acoustic meatus

C. Review of Landmarks and Positioning Lines (used for sinuses, mastoids, and temporal bone)

Locate the following on another person.

___ 1. Interpupillary line

___ 2. Midsagittal plane

___ 3. Canthus

___ 4. EAM

___ 5. Orbitomeatal line

___ 6. Nasion

___ 7. Mentomeatal line

___ 8. Acanthion

___ 9. Infraorbitomeatal line

___ 10. Mandibular symphysis

___ 11. Mastoid tip

___ 12. Superciliary arch

D. Film Critique and Evaluation

Your instructor will provide various radiographs of the basic and optional projections of the facial bones as described in this chapter. Some will be optimal quality radiographs meeting all or most of the evaluation criteria described for each projection in the textbook and/or audiovisuals. Others will be less than optimal quality and several will be unacceptable, requiring a repeat exam. Evaluate each radiograph as specified below.

Place a check by each of the following when it is completed.

___ 1. Critique each radiograph based on evaluation criteria provided for each projection in the textbook and/or audio-visuals. The following criteria guidelines can be used and checked as each radiograph is evaluated. (Additional checks can be placed to the left for each criteria guideline if more than six radiographs are evaluated.)

Radiographs 1 2 3 4 5 6	Criteria Guidelines
___ ___ ___ ___ ___ ___	a. Correct film size and correct orientation of part to film?
___ ___ ___ ___ ___ ___	b. Correct alignment and/or centering of part to film?
___ ___ ___ ___ ___ ___	c. Correct collimation and CR location?
___ ___ ___ ___ ___ ___	d. Pertinent anatomy well visualized?
___ ___ ___ ___ ___ ___	e. Motion?
___ ___ ___ ___ ___ ___	f. Optimum exposure; density and/or contrast?
___ ___ ___ ___ ___ ___	g. Patient ID information and markers?

___ 2. Based on acceptable variances to criteria factors, determine which of these radiographs are acceptable and which are unacceptable and should have been repeated.

Important: It is important that you have successfully carried out all of the exercises described above before taking the self-test and before going to your instructor for the chapter evaluation exam. If you neglect these exercises, you will not be able to meet all the objectives for this chapter and may not receive a passing grade for this course.

Answers to Review Exercise A

1. A. Frontal, usually two
    B. Ethmoid, many
    C. Sphenoid, one or two
    D. Maxillary, two

    E. Frontal
    F. Ethmoid
    G. Sphenoid
    H. Maxillary

2. Antrum or Antrum of Highmore

3. superior

4. (a) lateral masses or labyrinths
    (b) ethmoid

5. (a) body   (b) sphenoid

6. A. false (frontal sinuses rarely become
    aerated before age six)
    B. true
    C. false (usually comprised of three groups)
    D. true
    E. true
    F. false (this occurs in the maxillary
    sinuses, not frontal)
    G. true

7. A. Auricle or pinna
    B. External acoustic meatus
    C. Drum crest or spur
    D. Auditory ossicles
    E. Epitympanic recess or attic
    F. Semicircular canals
    G. Internal acoustic meatus
    H. Tympanic cavity
    I. Cochlea
    J. Eustachian or auditory tube
    K. Styloid process
    L. Mastoid process or tip

    M. Malleus
    N. Incus
    O. Stapes

    P. External acoustic meatus (may also have
    been identified as the tympanic
    membrane)
    Q. Stapes
    R. Incus
    S. Malleus
    T. Anterior
    U. Posterior

8. A. Posterior semicircular canal
    B. Lateral semicircular canal
    C. Superior semicircular canal
    D. Oval or vestibular window
    E. Vestibule
    F. Cochlea
    G. Round or cochlear window
    H. Anterior
    I. Posterior

9. A. Osseous labyrinth
    B. Membranous labyrinth

10. (a) cochlea   (b) semicircular canals

11. A. 10
    B. 1 to 1.5
    C. 14
    D. 9
    E. 5

If you missed more than 12 blanks, you should review this section again in the textbook and/or audio-visuals before continuing.

Answers to Review Exercise B

1. A. Frontal
    B. Maxillary
    C. Sphenoid

2. To demonstrate air-fluid levels

3. A. Lateral
    B. PA (Caldwell)
    C. Parietoacanthial (Waters)
    D. Submentovertex (SMV or basilar)

4. Axial transoral (open-mouth Waters)

5. A. Interpupillary line (IPL)
    B. Orbitomeatal line (OML)
    C. Mentomeatal line (MML)

6. A. Acanthion
    B. Nasion
    C. Midway between outer canthus and
        external acoustic meatus

7. sphenoid

8. A. Axiolateral oblique (Law method)
    B. Posterior profile or anterior oblique
        (Stenvers method)

9. A. AP axial (Towne method)
    B. Axioposterior oblique (Mayer method)

10. cartilage of auricle might superimpose
    mastoid air cells

11. (a) parallel (b) 45 (c) 12 (d) cephalic

12. down-side

13. bilateral

14. (a) down-side (b) 1 inch posterior to EAM

15. Posterior profile position (Stenvers method)

16. A. AP axial (Towne method)
    B. Submentovertex (SMV or basilar)

17. tomography

18. A. Ossicles
    B. Tympanic cavity
    C. Ossicles

19. A. Ossicles
    B. Cochlea
    C. External acoustic canal

If you missed more than 8 blanks, you should
review this section again in the textbook and/or
audio-visuals before continuing.

Self-Test

My score = _____ %

Directions: Take this self-test only after completing all the review exercises and laboratory activities in this chapter. Complete directions including grading requirements are described in the front pages of this workbook and in the self-test of Chapter 1.

Test

There are 75 blanks. Each correct blank is worth 1.3 points. (Spelling is important so correct any misspellings as you grade your test.)

1. Antrum of Highmore refers to the _maxillary_ sinuses.

2. The sphenoid sinus lies in the body of the (a) _sphenoid_ bone directly below the (b) _____
    sella turcica .

3. The ethmoid sinuses are usually arranged into (a) _three_ [anterior - middle - posterior] groups and are contained in the
    (b) _lateral masses_ of the (c) _ethmoid_ bone.
    (labyrinths)

4. The pars petrosa portion of the temporal bone is also commonly called the (a) _petrous pyramid_,
    the upper border of which is called the (b) _petrous ridge_ .

5. The three main portions of the temporal bone are:

    A. _squamous_

    B. _mastoid_

    C. _petrous_

6. Which of the above portions of the temporal bone house the organs of hearing? (a) _petrous_ ,
    Which houses the organs of equilibrium? (b) _petrous_ .

7. The three divisions of the ear are: (a) _external_ , (b) _middle_ , (c) _internal_.

8. The opening through the internal portion of the petrous pyramids which is important radiographically is
    called the (a) _internal acoustic meatus_. What structures pass through this opening?
    (b) _nerves + blood vessels_

9. Fill in the correct anatomical term for the following:

    A. External flap-like structure of ear _auricle (pinna)_

    B. Small, lip-like structure located anterior to ear opening _tragus_

    C. Ear drum _tympanic membrane_

    D. The sharp small bony projection to which the upper ear drum is attached (a) _drum crest (sp_

    which separates the external auditory meatus from the cavity called the (b) _____
    epitympanic recess (attic)

    E. The cavity directly inside the ear drum _tympanic cavity_

    F. Tube-like structure between middle ear and nasopharynx (a) _eustachian tube_,
    which is approximately (b) _4_ cm long. (auditory tube)

    G. The posterior communication of the mastoid air cells with the epitympanic recess or attic is through
    the _aditus_.

    H. The "large" chamber directly posterior to the above opening is the _antrum_.

    I. The auditory ossicle shaped like a stirrup is called the (a) _stapes_ and is attached to a mem-
    brane called the (b) _oval_ or (c) _vestibular_ window.

    J. The ossicle attached to the ear drum is the _malleus_.

    K. The ossicle shaped like a pre-molar tooth is the _incus_.

    L. The anterior portion of the osseous labyrinth is the ~~stapes~~ cochlea

    M. The middle portion of the osseous labyrinth is the ~~incus~~ vestibule

    N. The posterior portion of the osseous labyrinth includes the _semicircular canals_

    O. The (a) _oval (vestibular)_ window receives vibrations from the external ear through
    the (b) _stapes_.

    P. The (a) _round_ or (b) _cochlear_ window is located at the base of the
    first coil of the cochlea which is covered by a membrane which allows movements of the non-
    compressible fluid inside the closed duct system of the membranous labyrinth.

10. The TEA is an external landmark corresponding to approximately what important internal structure?
    petrous ridges

11. The external acoustic meatus is approximately _2.5_ cm long.

12. What basic mastoid projection or position will best visualize the bony labyrinths and the internal acoustic
    canal? _anterior oblique (Stenvers)_

13. The three important divisions of the osseous labyrinth are:

    A. _cochlea_   hearing

    B. _vestibule_

    C. _semicircular canals_   equilibrium

14. A. Which of the above houses the organs of hearing? _cochlea_

    B. Which houses the organs of equilibrium? _semicircular canals_

15. Fill in the following distances on an average shaped skull.

    A. Back of head to mid EAM _10_ cm

         table top IAM → 9
         IAM – EAM (outh) 5 / 14

    Lateral measurements (to side away from table top)

    B. Table top to internal acoustic meatus _8 9_ cm   5→EAM to EAM

         table to drum crest 11.5
         EAM   2.5 / 14.0

    C. Table top to auditory ossicles _11–11.5_ cm

    D. Table top to area of tympanic membrane or drum crest or spur _11.5_ cm

16. A routine paranasal sinus series should include the following four projections or positions.

    A. _lateral_

    B. _PA (Caldwell)_

    C. _parietoacanthial (Waters)_

    D. _Submentovertex (basilar)_

17. Which of the routine sinus projections best demonstrates the sphenoid sinus? _lateral_

18. Which of the routine sinus projections best demonstrates the maxillary sinuses? _Waters_

19. Which of the routine sinus projections best demonstrates the frontal sinuses? _Caldwell_

20. Why must sinus radiography be done erect and with a horizontal x-ray beam? _to show_ _air-fluid levels_

21. In the posterior profile or Stenver's position with the right side of the face toward the table, which petrous pyramid will be radiographed? _Side down right_

22. What is the centering point (part placed to center of film) or the CR location on the following projections/positions for demonstrating the paranasal sinuses:

    A. Axial transoral (open-mouth Waters) _acanthion_

    B. Submentovertex _1.5 in. below mandibular symphysis_

    C. Lateral _midway between outer canthus + EAM_

    D. PA (Caldwell) _nasion_

    E. Parietoacanthial (Waters) _acanthion_

     9.5 – 10.5 – tomos middle ear
     9.9 IAM

23. Which positioning line is perpendicular to the plane of the film on the following: (Use abbreviations or initials.)

A. Posterior profile (Stenvers) _____IOML_____

B. AP axial (Towne) _____OML_____

C. Axioposterior oblique (Mayer) _____IOML_____

D. Lateral sinuses _____IPL_____

E. PA (Caldwell) _____OML_____

F. Parietoacanthial (Waters) _____MML_____ mentomeatal

24. The two most common basic projections/position for the mastoids are:

A. _____axiolateral (Law)_____

B. _____anterior oblique (Stenvers)_____

25. Air-fluid levels in the _____sphenoid_____ sinuses may be evidence of a basilar skull fracture.

Answers to Self-Test

1. maxillary

2. (a) sphenoid   (b) sella turcica

3. (a) three   (b) lateral masses or labyrinths
   (c) ethmoid

4. (a) petrous portion, or petrous pyramid
   (b) petrous ridge

5. A. Squamous portion
   B. Mastoid portion
   C. Petrous portion

6. (a) petrous portion   (b) petrous portion

7. (a) external   (b) middle   (c) internal

8. (a) internal acoustic meatus   (b) certain
   nerves and blood vessels

9. A. Auricle of pinna
   B. Tragus
   C. Tympanic membrane
   D. (a) drum crest or spur
      (b) epitympanic recess or attic
   E. Tympanic cavity
   F. (a) eustachian or auditory tube   (b) 4
   G. aditus
   H. antrum
   I. (a) stapes   (b) oval   (c) vestibular
   J. malleus
   K. incus
   L. cochlea
   M. vestibule
   N. semicircular canals
   O. (a) oval or vestibular   (b) stapes
   P. (a) round   (b) cochlea

10. Lateral portion of petrous ridge

11. 2.5

12. Posterior profile (Stenvers)

13. A. Cochlea
    B. Vestibule
    C. Semicircular canals

14. A. Cochlea
    B. Semicircular canals

15. A. 10
    B. 9
    C. 11 to 11.5
    D. 11.5

16. A. Lateral
    B. PA Caldwell
    C. Parietoacanthial
    D. Submentovertex

17. Lateral

18. Waters

19. PA Caldwell

20. To demonstrate air-fluid levels

21. Right

22. A. Acanthion
    B. CR midway between angles of mandible
       1.5 inches inferior to mandibular
       symphysis
    C. Midway between outer canthus and
       external acoustic meatus
    D. Nasion
    E. Acanthion

23. A. IOML
    B. OML
    C. IOML
    D. IPL
    E. OML
    F. MML

24. A. Axiolateral oblique (Law)
    B. Posterior profile (Stenvers)

25. sphenoid